SOUND *of* SILENCE

'And in the naked light I saw,
Ten thousand people, maybe more.
People talking without speaking,
People hearing without listening'

Paul Simon and Art Garfunkel, 1966

When communication fails, there is only silence

This book is for my father, who was deaf, my mother, who lived with a deaf man, my husband John, who supports my work, my wonderful children, for whom I was away so much, and to Peter Blamey, my business partner and friend.

SOUND *of* SILENCE

DR ELAINE SAUNDERS

CONTENTS

Preface   5

School nanny at 16 – My experience of deaf education   8

Becoming an audiologist   26

Working in trendy Fulham in the '70s   46

How we hear, what can go wrong

    and how hearing changes your brain   54

How well can you hear?   73

The sound of trees, the noise of trains   82

My dad; running, boating and hearing   94

Ice-creams and hearing tests   102

I've come to look for America   116

Transportation to Elysium Fields   132

The curl at the end of the electrode   137

Just like winning the lottery…   157

From then to now – the changing look and sound

    of hearing aids   162

Hearing dynamically – the next big thing in hearing aids   184

My own hearing aid company, and much more, at last   199

Blamey Saunders hears – a revolution in hearing aid service   211

To hear or not to hear: That wasn't a question…   225

People hearing without listening   236

Afterthought   245

PREFACE

In 1886, Dr William R Roe, the headmaster and Founder of the Deaf and Dumb asylum in Derby (later the Derby School for the Deaf) wrote a book that he called *Anecdotes and Incidents of the Deaf and Dumb*. In the book, he tells the story of Jim, who was misunderstood and treated as mentally deficient. Roe tells us that a man, who said his name was Jim, was found wandering about in a strange manner at the local railway station. He was subsequently charged at the local police court, with being 'a wandering lunatic'. The police sergeant who had found him also ascertained that the man had come from Bath. It's not a particularly straightforward railway trip from Bath to Derby. Apparently, he had similarly been found wandering around at the railway station in Bath. The sergeant, in Derby, talked to Jim, and decided that Jim in fact wanted to go to London, but the Sergeant couldn't persuade him to buy a ticket to London. Jim only had a few possessions with him. He had a basket, containing some tea, a razor and other small articles; but no letters or anything from which they could find where he wanted to go. Jim continued to be held in the police cells. The police surgeon examined him and 'pronounced him to be of unsound mind'. Someone, perhaps the perspicuous police sergeant, had the wit to send for William Roe, the town expert on deafness.

Mr. Roe, communicated with the prisoner using sign language, and found that Jim 'was deaf and dumb, and totally uneducated, but certainly of sound mind'. Jim was released into Roe's care, and the whole story emerged

5

over the next few days. It turned out that Jim had been staying with a friend in Bath, and had wanted to visit some other friends across town. He went to the train station in Bath, and the railway authorities decided, mistakenly, that Jim wanted to go to Derby, and put him on a train to Derby. Jim was understandably somewhat confused.

There wasn't a lot of awareness or understanding of deafness in the 1880s. But would the situation be better if this had happened today? I fear it might not be. Perhaps we are more caring today, which means authorities may have acted even sooner to over organise Jim, be it with the best intentions. But children with deafness or hearing loss are still misdiagnosed or not detected in most developed countries today. The head of the International Rotary Action Group on hearing, Ellen Haggerty, an energised and very intelligent, severely deaf person, has had the experience of being treated in a rather patronising manner, and over organised by other people. Even in circumstances of good intention, actions can be patronising, controlling and misguided.

Today I part own a small international hearing aid company that's changing the world of hearing aids forever. I'm working with clever scientists to use the world of the Internet to deliver a new kind of hearing aid straight to the home, wherever people are, and at much lower costs than are usually associated with high quality hearing aids. The hearing aid, based on bionic ear technology is very, very good, but we have made it so simple that people can take control and set it up themselves. My goal is to help people hear better, and to live easier lives.

Untreated hearing loss, when acquired as an adult, even if it's not severe, can have a big negative impact on people lives. It's a cause of depression, paranoia, deteriorating relationships, disadvantages in the work place and even early cognitive decline. I'm trying to help, by raising awareness, working with clever people on new technologies and helping people take control of their hearing themselves. I believe that many hearing aids are overpriced, and many don't work very well. This is my story, which starts about the time that Simon and Garfunkel's enduring song was released, a story to try and overcome the silence. The reader will learn about hearing, listening, what can go wrong, what can be done and some moving stories from people, including my father, who have triumphed over their hearing problems. My path has taken me from being a lowly assistant in a school for deaf children, through the development of the cochlear implant to leading a very new kind of hearing aid company in Australia.

Hearing and listening helps keep the brain fit. This book could have been called – 'How Hearing Changes your Brain'. In the pages ahead, my story will mingle with strategies to keep people's hearing fitter and more useful to overall health.

CHAPTER ONE

SCHOOL NANNY AT 16 – MY EXPERIENCE OF DEAF EDUCATION

' If you want to win something, run 100 meters. If you want to
experience something, run a marathon. '
- Emil Zatopek, 1952 Olympic Marathon gold medalist

I trained and competed as a 400-metre track runner. I learned a lot of discipline. Believe it or not, the 400 meters does require some strategic thinking, even though it's over quickly. But, if you are determined to fulfil your dream, you may need strategy, combined with the skills of a marathon runner. My father was deaf and he wasn't a big talker. It may have been partly because of his deafness and his need to adapt his communication style to accommodate his deafness. It may just have been his personality. He was, after all, an engineer, and tended to be a man of action and creativity rather than a storyteller. What was cause, and what was effect? I don't know. Dad was a civil engineer, analytic, disliked the 'airy fairy', and didn't suffer fools very gladly. Nor do I. Like father, like daughter. He planned and managed railways for a living. In Derby, England, where we moved from London to live when I was nine, your Dad either worked for the railway or for Rolls Royce Ltd. My Dad, even with poor hearing, had a very senior role in British Rail. He led successful project teams and he travelled a lot. He did a management course before they were trendy, and told me that making a strategic plan for your life was probably impossible. You have to take opportunities and be prepared for the unexpected. At this stage I agree. It's easy to look back and identify some kind of pattern, but it would be the unusual person who didn't find bumps in the road.

My father became the founding Chairman of the Friends of the Royal School for the Deaf in Derby. The role ranged from the strategic to the very practical. One of his duties became to drive some of the schoolboys to cub scouts, with me in the passenger seat trying to keep order. My Dad wasn't always deaf. His hearing started to get muffled and then disappeared. He had otosclerosis. This is sometimes called 'arthritis of the ear' where the bones in the middle ear fuse together, causing hearing loss. Eventually, the bony growth grows into the sensory part of the ear causing permanent hearing loss. Otosclerosis is sometimes known as Beethoven's Deafness. Beethoven has helped us understand what he and others who suffered from otosclerosis experienced, He started to lose his hearing in his mid twenties, which is common for otosclerosis. He left us some insights into his personal experience of deafness in the letters that he wrote: 'For two years, I have avoided almost all social gatherings, because it is impossible for me to say to people, I am deaf.' Thus Beethoven's voice comes through the years, and many thousands of people have found themselves in the same situation of trying to cover up their hearing difficulty, or simply avoiding social events. Beethoven looked for cures. He wrote a letter to his childhood friend and physician, Franz Wegeler, to tell him that he had read about a deaf child who experienced restored hearing after being treated by 'galvanism'. Galvanism, was named after Luigi Galvani, by Antonio Volta. It describes the contraction of a muscle that has been stimulated by an electric current. Italian physician Luigi Galvani noticed on a summer's day in 1786 muscular spasms in dead frog's legs suspended by copper hooks from an iron bar. He called the effect, 'animal electricity'. The word galvanism refers to any form of medical treatment involving the application of pulses of electric current to body tissues provoking the contraction of muscles that are stimulated by the electric current. It implied the release, through electricity, of mysterious life forces to the dead. Galvanism and the occult were the inspiration for Mary Shelley's horror story *Frankenstein*. In the preface to *Frankenstein*, she wrote, 'I saw the hideous phantasm of a man stretched out, and then, on the working of some powerful engine, show signs of life, and stir…' We don't know whether or not Beethoven pursued this cure, but if he did then it didn't work, and he later wrote: 'From year to year, my hopes of being cured have gradually been shattered.' Today if 'Beethoven's deafness', or otosclerosis, is caught early, it can be corrected by surgery. My father had an operation, but the condition was too far progressed, and he lost most of his hearing.

The famous 18th century artist, Sir Joshua Reynolds, by contrast, a man who depended on a visual interpretation of the world, considered that his deafness sharpened his interpretation of the world and enhanced his art. The fact that he painted himself with a cupped hand at his ear, to demonstrate his deafness, indicates the degree to which he had embraced it.

I grew up knowing that I had to make my tiny contribution to making the world a better place, whatever I did in life. Aware of this, my father encouraged me to take on volunteer work at the residential School for the Deaf in Derby. In his role as Chairman of the League of Friends, coupled with his own experiences, he had come to understand some of the challenges that the children there faced. In a residential school their challenges included being tucked away from family life. My father wanted more opportunities and more normality for the children, and thought that I might be able to use my Saturdays to help out. I was inspired to help, if somewhat naïve about my limitations.

One rainy Saturday, I turned up for my first full day volunteering at the school. I walked up the steps of a very imposing building and through heavy, dark brown, double doors. I was sixteen.

The school looked Dickensian, both inside and out, proclaiming its age. It was founded as a charity in 1892 by William Roe and opened in 1897 after a £12,000 fund-raising push. Pupils learned practical skills, and the three R's, (Reading, (w)Riting and (a)Rithmetic). The curriculum was otherwise narrow. The boys were instructed in carpentry, metalwork, boot repairing and gardening, while the girls were taught cookery and laundry work. Dr Roe had initially been inspired to dedicate his life to helping deaf people after meeting a young deaf man called Jack. The young William Roe was struck by how miserably people treated Jack. That was in an era when the effects of deafness weren't really understood, and deaf education was understood even less. Dr Roe's first school opened two years later, in 1894, in Belper, which is a small town, not far from Derby. When the school in Belper first opened, it only had 16 students. Dr Roe was Headmaster and his wife, Lydia, became a teacher there. She was the first woman in England who qualified to teach deaf children, and left a legacy of a book, *The Teaching of Language During the Early Period of a Deaf Child's School Life.*

The school moved to elegant Friargate, near the Great Northern railway station in Derby, in 1897, where they were able to build an imposing building complex, little of which remains today.

William Roe's school was very progressive for its time. He used to take his children out on road shows to show his methods of education. The following extract from the Buxton Advertiser in September, 1884 tells of an exhibition they gave in the Peak District town of Buxton.

'The Entertainments given on Tuesday in the Pavilion by Deaf and Dumb children from the Institution at Derby drew large audiences. The

children looked bright and happy, and their personal appearance was a sufficient indication that they were taken good care of at the Institution. Mr. Roe gave some interesting illustrations of teaching the dumb to speak on the oral system by placing the youngest girl on a chair and explaining how sounds were produced. Mr. Roe asked various questions as to names and objects orally, to which answers were instantly given in the same way. The Institution at Derby is an excellent one, and the Committee of management deserve the warmest thanks for what has already been achieved, and we hope will be materially assisted in north Derbyshire by all Christian people...'

It was to the original complex of buildings, built by Roe, that I was entering more than 70 years later. Most of the original buildings were pulled down in 1974, although a fine old Queen Anne house that formed part of the complex remains. Today, the Royal School for the Deaf, is housed in attractive buildings, suitable for modern teaching methods, and equipped with the latest technology. Children come to Derby from all over England to attend the school, and the progressive education includes teaching British Sign Language.

However, in the late 1960s, a period generally known for its bright colours, and extensive use of chrome and plastic, I thought the place looked dreary. I remember lots of Institutional Green. That's a real name for a colour – a sort of greyish green that was common in hospitals, government buildings, and other institutions, which is how it earned its name. An authoritative, but matronly woman who I later came to really admire and like, as the head House Mother, showed me into the 'Day Room'. There were two scuffed couches pushed against each sidewall and a low formica coffee table with a lamp on it. A few children milled around, glancing out the window as they moved from the couch to the coffee table, and generally ignored me. I thought they must mostly be about seven or eight years old. The lady who met me at the door, the weekend duty house mother, told me that she much preferred to see the children go home at weekends. But there were several children who rarely, if ever, went home at weekends. She told me that some of the parents were embarrassed by their imperfect children, and didn't know what to do with them, so the children stayed at the school all term, and didn't go home at weekends. The House Mother said that sometimes the reason lay in the family's cultural background, but she thought that sometimes it was just that, as parents, they really didn't know what to do. But the school had little in the way of plans and activities for the weekend as the teachers had gone home.

It was here that I met Donald. Donald was an amazing West Indian kid, about seven years old, whose parents didn't want anyone to know he was deaf, so Donald would stay at school on weekends. Though I was a passionate volunteer, it was also a Saturday and I was a teenager. I wanted to go out with my friends, and so Donald used to come with me to the coffee bar. The Kardomah Cafe was the place to be on a Saturday afternoon in Derby.

This was the fashionable late 60s: flowing clothes and Afghan coats, flowery smocks, bell bottom jeans and men with long hair, or Beatles haircuts. At the Kardomah there was plenty of music and probably lots of tobacco smoke, although I never smoked. Donald would trail along for his Saturday afternoon milkshake, and was very patient being taken around by me, a well-meaning but somewhat inept volunteer. I would usually then take him to watch my friend play hockey in the Derby 1st team and he would be very absorbed in the game. Sometimes we went to the football, with some of the other older boys in the school, to see Derby County. We went in a minibus, were ushered to priority seats and didn't have to queue up or stand to watch the game.

Donald was very deaf. There were no cochlear implants yet, and his hearing aids were not up to much. He wasn't allowed to sign at school, so he didn't know any formal sign language. Lydia's teaching legacy advised teachers to hold their hands behind their backs to avoid gestures. And yet Donald was extremely engaging, with very expressive eyes that he used to good effect in his communication. He must have developed that from an early age. Like all the children in the school, he made good use of gesture when no one was looking. My friends loved him, and his off-beat humour, and the hockey team that we went to watch came to depend on him being there. Meaningful, communicative friendships were built in silence, each Saturday at the cafe and a sporting field. I have long since lost touch with Donald and wonder what happened to him. Perhaps he had a good time with us. I hope so. I was trying to 'do good', and it was probably better than sitting in the Day Room at school, but I dragged this poor kid everywhere that I wanted to go on a teenagers afternoon out in the 60s in Derby.

As a teenager, I didn't realise that I was entering Deaf Education at a time of controversy and change. Deaf education in 1969 had more in common with the 1850s than with the 1990s. All I knew then was that these children couldn't hear, and as a result were stuck in this horrible old building, with no family, at weekends. In the 1880s most teachers used sign language to teach deaf children. But things changed and it became the trend to teach children through the spoken word, which we call oral/aural education. This literally means a form of education involving talking and hearing. The problem was that the children couldn't hear, so it was a rather inadequate form of oral/aural education. In fact, a report published as late as the 1970s showed that deaf children leaving school at 16 generally had a reading age of less than ten. Pure oralism, that is education using the voice, was not the great success that its early proponents had hoped. Language and speech was the only focus, and took most of the time, and so the education curriculum was very narrow. It makes me think how much we rely on language, in whatever form. Listen to Lydia Roe, whose writings give us insights to the state of the art in the late 1800s.

'A great impetus may be given to language teaching if slips of paper with all newly acquired sounds, words, phrases or sentences written on, be given to each child as they are taught in class for in most day rooms there are blackboards or slates, and nothing pleases the little ones more than playing at school. The slips of paper would be treasured because a teacher had given them, and the work would go on continuously...'

For centuries there had been debate in education about oralism versus manualism, which is education using the voice versus using the hands. Educators were polarised in their views. The response to a shocking 1970 report was for educators to diversify and try all sorts of different methods, but really they were still using much of the time trying to teach communication, rather than content or skills. This diversity didn't bring about the hoped for results. Many deaf young people came out of school unable to communicate with hearing people at all, or even with other deaf young people, especially if they had been to different schools. Frustrated children in oral schools made up their own local sign language to communicate with each other. This was the tragedy of the system – leaving children belonging to neither the deaf signing community, nor the hearing world. The history of deaf education is fascinating, but today it seems strange that we ever went through this educational evolution. There's an interesting philosophical book on language and deafness by Jonathon Rees, who in 1999 wrote:

'The story of deaf education has great lessons to teach us: the brutality of ignorant cruelty, the tenuousness of scientific progress and last, but not least, the stubborn persistence of folk metaphysics.'

I fear that all of these things still haunt education and health science today.

William Roe was a leader although stories of his time seem against today's knowledge. In his book, *Anecdotes of the Deaf and Dumb*, he printed a letter that he had received in the early days of the institution:

'*A lady writes about a little boy she had assisted in obtaining admission into the Institution, and said that "During the little time (18 months) that William has been in the Institution he has improved wonderfully." She writes – "You know he used to be so wild, dirty, and careless; he was always interfering with everybody, in fact he went in the village by the name of Troublesome Dummy. All is changed; he is a nice clean, well-behaved boy, and people are beginning to call him by his right name, William. We shall never forget what you have done for him."*'

This reflects, not so much Roe's teaching as his advocacy in raising awareness of hearing loss and changing attitudes.

Much of what we take for granted today about individuality, and the nature of disability, was actually quite recent. In fact, it was at the 21st International Congress on the Education of the Deaf in 2010, in Vancouver, that a statement was released, including an apology, to reverse the dictate of the 1880 Milan conference in which sign language was officially banned from deaf education.

The 17th century physician, John Bulwer, was the first Englishman to develop a method for communicating with the deaf and dumb and was the first to recommend the institution of 'an academy of the mute', but it was the French Abbé Charles-Michel de l'Épée, who lived in Paris in the 1700s who is recorded as the major figure in the history of sign language. He founded a free public school for deaf children in Paris in 1760, called the Nationale de Sourds-Muéts Institution and there he began to develop a system of sign language and instruction, which eventually became an educational method based on gestures. He sensibly learned the gestures from the children themselves, and incorporated them into signing. Then he worked out how to translate that into written French. The Abbé was not starting from scratch. He knew that there was already a signing deaf community in Paris using what was known as 'Old French Sign Language', but he thought that their language was primitive and could be improved to give scope for written French. The hearing teachers at his school were taught to use the Old French Sign Language with their students. Because he had based his work on the gestures that the children were already using, he was able to 'make official' the incumbent vernacular. When the teachers were formally instructing the children in the classroom, they used the combination of the Abbé's idiosyncratic gestural system and other invented signs to represent all the verb endings, articles, prepositions, and auxiliary verbs of the French language. This became the basis of many sign languages, including signed English. Today, we write English more or less as we say it. The Abbé was trying to take that step with sign language, whilst also expanding the gestural lexicon. Essentially, he was incorporating finger spelling.

Other paths were being explored in Scotland at about the same time. The gifted teacher, Thomas Braidwood, was also championing a gesture based communication method. He established the first school for the deaf in Edinburgh, Braidwood's Academy for the Deaf and Dumb. Braidwood's Academy was a private school, in more than one sense of this term, as Thomas Braidwood was rather secretive about his teaching methods. Although the signing component, known as the Braidwoodian method, which combined sign with finger spelling, like the Abbé, is generally accepted was the forerunner of British Sign Language and recognized as a language in its own right in 2003, Braidwood's overall method, was to combine speaking with his gesture and finger spelling based sign language, to create an educational method similar to what we today call 'The Total Communication Method', where signing and oralism are used together.

The scene was being assembled for debate on different methods of deaf education. This was a big step from the status quo of no education for deaf children. In Germany, ex-military man, Samuel Heinicke, was developing a method that combined a speaking/hearing approach with finger spelling. He was very passionate about his methods, and he kept up a robust correspondence with his rival, the French Abbé. Heinicke started tutoring in 1754, but founded his own school in 1777, which is an active school today. The school's original name was the 'Electoral Saxon Institute for Mutes and Other Persons Afflicted with Speech Defects', and today it is known as the 'Samuel Heinicke School for the Deaf'. He taught speech by having students feel the throat. Heinicke wrote about his use of speech to teach deaf students and dubbed it 'Oralism'. His methods became known as 'The German Method', but it was still not pure oralism, being coupled with finger spelling. In this climate of debate, oralism seemed to be winning. However, influenced by Abbé de l'Épée's successor, Abbé Sicard, Thomas Hopkins Gallaudet began a sign-language institution for the deaf in the USA, which is thriving today, as both a school and a University.

'The Total Communication' style of teaching, adopted by Heinicke and Braidwood, became strictly oral when Heinicke's son-in-law, Carl Reich, became the head teacher of the Leibnitz school. Reich banned both signing and finger-spelling, an approach which was to be carried forward into the late 20th century.

The oral path was prominently followed by the famous Alexander Graham Bell, himself the son of a deaf mother, and whose father and grandfather were both elocutionists; teachers who specialised in speech articulation and delivery. Alexander Graham Bell's father pioneered what he called 'Visible Speech', which was a system of symbols to assist people in articulation in any language. It's basically a phonetic alphabet, but is also known as the Physiologic Alphabet, because of the classification that is based on articulation. Alexander Bell became a teacher to deaf children, but developed his own system of teaching, using a combination of speech and lip-reading. Bell strongly believed that oral education would make it easier for deaf and hearing people to mix. He took this very literally into the school system, and was an early visionary in the area of integrated education. He proposed that small groups of deaf children would be taught alongside hearing children in day schools, differing from the predominantly residential approach. He was successful in establishing these units in several states in the USA. Other than this far-sighted move he had some interesting ideas that today we would find unacceptably discriminatory. Oral education was very difficult without good hearing aids, so oral schools sometimes continued the draconian tradition in forbidding children to sign at all. The oralist movement thought this would lead to better integration at school and continued to uphold Bell's ideas of integrated education.

There have been many political, philosophical and religious influences on deaf education, and there are whole books devoted to the topic. The history of deaf education lies in three broad phases, and for all the formal debate, the successes were probably due to the different educators' confidence and teaching abilities, rather than their methods. Was it the teacher, or was it the method? This is a question that can be applied to educational methods as far apart as Montessori and Steiner education. Sometimes, great educators or therapists are confused in history with the methods they used. The methods are then copied; the success rate is not. Initially, deaf education was about teaching children to sign so they could learn about the world, and religion. Then education became oral, as in talking, but not really 'aural', as they couldn't hear, so that children could be part of the hearing world. Aural/Oralism became the end in itself, rather than a means to a rounded education. But the trouble is, humans have a need to communicate, so if you can't hear, then signing seemed more natural. Children found it much easier to express themselves that way. Today, young children who have normal hearing are sometimes taught to sign as it is a faster way for them to be able to express themselves, before their fine motor skills have mastered the complex articulation processes of speech. It's thought to reduce frustration, and hence take the 'terrible' out of 'twos'.

Given that I went on to study audiology at the University of Manchester, I'll put the spotlight on Sir Alexander and Lady Ewing, who founded the department of Audiology and Deaf Education there, and who had a great influence on the education of deaf children through the 20th century. Professor Alexander Ewing, who was knighted for his work in audiology in 1958, was based at Manchester University from 1915 until the 1960s. Professor Ewing's close professional colleague and soon to be wife, Irene Rosetta Goldsack, had been appointed as the first lecturer in deaf education on the Diploma of Deaf Education, which had been established at Manchester University. The opportunity came about thanks to a legacy from the family of a profoundly deaf young man Ellis Llwyd Jones, who died in 1918. His wealthy father, Sir James Jones, donated a substantial sum of money to the University of Manchester in order to establish the first university-based programme for teachers of the deaf, and also to carry out research into childhood deafness. As a direct result of this legacy, the University of Manchester established a lectureship for training teachers of the deaf on the oral method of teaching in 1919. The fact that training was exclusively oral severed any possibility of a link between deaf adults using sign and the education of deaf children. The gap between what educators thought and promoted started to move further and further from the views of the deaf community – a rift that has not been fully bridged today.

The Ewings wrote a comprehensive account of their beliefs and methodology in a book entitled *Speech and the Deaf Child* (1954). In it they detail the three essential conditions of speech intelligibility – understanding, skill and practice – stating that none of these could be acquired by children on their own without the constant help of sympathetic, knowledgeable and skillful teachers. Their methodology relied heavily on the use of residual hearing.

Oral education had a terrible disadvantage until the advent of good hearing aids and cochlear implants. Hearing aids weren't commonly used in oral education until about the 1940s, and even then they didn't work very well. Despite that, over the next fifteen to twenty years, opinion became established that hearing aids helped the hearing of deaf children enough for education to become truly aural/oral. Children began to gain access to audiology services, and their hearing loss could be quantified in relation to people with normal hearing. After the invention of the audiometer, children were asked to listen to the softest pure tones that they could hear. It did not give much insight into the type of hearing problems the children had, but it did give some guide to how much hearing loss they had, compared to children with good hearing.

Hearing aids at this time were large and typically worn in a harness, strapped to a child's front or back. The sound processing was rather simple. The hearing aids just made sounds louder which, it is now known, is not all that's needed. The hearing aids generally had a fairly large amplifier connected by wires to a heavy separate battery pack and by a further wire to an earpiece. The hearing aid user was thoroughly 'wired up'. Adults, who arranged the child's hearing aid, often tucked the hearing aid into a clothes item for security. The child would have heard a lot of noise from clothes rubbing on the microphone. Older women were inclined to tuck their own hearing aid into their bra and then shake in the talcum powder. Men were luckier, and put them in their top pockets – and were less likely to use talcum powder. Because the microphone was on the top of the case of the main body worn piece, the 'ear' was effectively in the top pocket, or tucked between your breasts. Whilst children escaped the clothes noise, by using a harness, their effective ear was still somewhere odd. The hearing aids were quite often put in a harness on the child's back, so that their movement was not restricted. The problem was that the microphone then, was on the top of the hearing aid and hence on the child's back – hardly a good replicate for the human ear. So, deaf education moved into the oral era, and it was expected that children would use their hearing, but nobody really understood at that time what they were actually hearing.

It wasn't until the introduction of cochlear implants, and the recognition that children benefit from early implantation, that the situation changed. Today children who get a cochlear implant young are likely to develop such good oral language, that they can go through mainstream school. There are many spin offs from the development and use of cochlear implants which has helped us understand more about hearing and to develop better hearing aids. Educators became much more comfortable about allowing signing, once children could hear more, and so 'Total Communication' became normal, although possibly not for the right reasons. I couldn't have dreamt when I started out at the Royal School for the Deaf that I'd be doing what I do today. I knew I was going to do something to help in the field of hearing loss; I knew I was deeply moved by the frustration and challenges of the children that I worked with, but computers were in their infancy and very, very large, and the Internet was almost unknown and with limited access.

I experienced an environment and educational method, at the Royal School for the Deaf in Derby, that was a product of the thinking about deaf education at the time. But when I started, as a teenager, I knew nothing about education of the deaf, which was probably an advantage. I was open minded, and keen to help, and accepted the wisdom of my elders there. I had been brought up with values of kindness and compassion, and I probably took deafness for granted. I was never surprised, embarrassed or thought too much about whether or not someone could hear. I'd grown up with a deaf father, although apparently I was guilty of saying to my mother more than once, 'Why does Daddy say such funny things?' As I grew up, I realised that I had to be sure that Dad understood what was being said to him. How else was I going to get driven to the track training session, or get my pocket money? There were no gains to be had in playing 'hard to communicate'. I didn't see my dad as limited, as he was a successful man. My mother would tell a different story, and saw his struggles and disappointments. Rightly or wrongly, I don't remember ever giving him any sympathy in relation to his hearing loss, but I must have felt it at least a bit, to have spent my whole adult life trying to make life better for people who lose their hearing. I've grown up and older pushing to my limits, and perhaps I see that as normal. Although Derby was an oral school, they weren't as strict as some of the schools about not signing, but I don't remember them teaching signing either. So the language of the classroom was speech. The language of the playground was informal gesture and sign, and indeed it was very local. The word for headmaster at the Derby school was to run a finger down their arm. When they wore their uniform it had green stripes, the headmaster was Mr Green. Today, the children learn British Sign Language, and they no longer have green stripes as their uniform. I eventually became a full time employee as a teaching assistant and child care assistant on £5.00 a week. Even in 1971 this wasn't much money, and I didn't get paid at all in school holidays. But by then I thought I had found my career vocation and that I would become a Teacher of the Deaf. The work as a teaching assistant would be good experience, before I went to University. I was living at home, so the money didn't really matter too much. Today we would be shocked that the job was so little valued that it was acceptable to hire a totally unqualified 16 year old, on less than a living wage. During the school day, I was to be on breakfast duty, on playground duty, and usually on dinner and evening duty. Evening duty meant more playtime, bath time and bedtime. Most days I would also work as an assistant in the classroom for at least half a day.

My first day as a teaching assistant was memorable and not promising. Inside the large Victorian building, at the end of the long Institutional Green corridor upstairs, the primary teacher frowned as he searched his pockets. Eight children and I waited expectantly.

'Hang on' he mumbled, 'I've forgotten my key. Just wait here with them, I'll be right back.'

I nodded as he powered down the corridor and disappeared down the stairs. That was the moment when I realised, to full effect, that children who depend on lip reading do not 'hear' you if they are not looking at you. And with that, eight children, looked away from me and bolted down the long wide corridor and down the stairs. 'Come back!' I cried, weakly. Of course no one heard, and no one turned around to read my lips. It must have been a few minutes later, the teacher returned with eight children in tow. He'd rounded them up in the playground.

I could see that, for all my good intentions and intuition, my disadvantage was that I was quite young and inexperienced. I needed to maintain the order and routine that the children needed to advance through their education. I knew that the only way I would be able to harness this kind of control over the group of children was by building a rapport with each child as individuals, and hope that in turn these children would each maintain their focus on me for instructions and would behave for me out of a sense of personal loyalty. Dinner was a major event. The whole school would dine together at long refectory tables and there was a friendly looking fireplace. The children were usually very good-humoured with me most of the time, given that I wasn't much older than them. They knew they had the upper hand and that any control from me required them to look at me directly. So mostly, they didn't, and it was actually the occupation of eating dinner that provided a semblance of order. Then it was on to bath time. There were about 25 children housed in a separate building that had once been the Sanatorium, now known as Junior House. There were two of us on duty at any time and there were three of us on staff. We all shared a room, but as the newest person in, and the youngest, I just got a camp bed. At bath time, we bathed the children two at a time. The big clawfoot bath was in the centre of the room, making a production line easy. The children would make two long lines, one on each side of the bath, and got put in two at a time, one from each side. Then they'd hop out the other side to a waiting towel. It was a big, draughty, Victorian building. The children must have been cold, standing there, waiting for their turn. I remember a lot of laughing. I hope my memory is right.

CHAPTER TWO

Becoming an Audiologist

When I was at school in Derby in the 1960s, I had already decided that I wanted to make a difference to the lives of people who had partial hearing or deafness.

My Dad was a big influence in persuading me that to do anything worthwhile, I should first study science at University. He thought it was the best basis for any next steps. I wasn't sure then that he was right, but it turned out he was. My all-girls and somewhat old-fashioned school in Derby, England then had a head teacher, who thought it would be good to get some of 'her girls' into science. I'd studied the traditional trio of chemistry, physics and maths, and especially enjoyed chemistry. Then I discovered the sub-atomic world, and the excitement of exploring a field where we knew so little. I decided to study Chemical Physics, which is the branch of physics that studies chemical processes from the point of view of physics. It relies heavily on mathematics, and may be considered as on the border of philosophy too.

I decided to go to Manchester University, because they offered an Undergraduate degree in Chemical Physics. The topic investigates chemical properties using techniques from atomic and molecular physics which can assist us to find out the behaviour of unstable and volatile chemicals and chemical reactions.

I chose Manchester for none of the right reasons. It turned out to be a great choice, as I was able to stay in the same city to go onto study audiology, but here's my confession. There weren't many courses in Chemical Physics, which narrowed the field, and Manchester had a great athletics track, right beside a hall of residence – how good was that? The Hall, Owens Park, was what was then, considered to be a very progressive, mixed student village. On the day of my interview at the University, it was sunny, and a really nice, and very good-looking young researcher showed us round. Happily they offered me a place, at a time when only 3% of young people went to University. We remember a lot in our hearing memory. Mine, for my time in Manchester includes Cat Stevens, David Bowie, Queen, Dr Feelgood, Ralph McTell and The Who – not forgetting the Halle Orchestra, of course.

Before I went to University I had another adventure, which evoked some strong sound memories. Our memory is shaped by auditory experiences as well as visual. Before I went to University, I had saved up enough money to go to the Olympic Games in Munich. I went on a package tour with a school, where some of the students had dropped out, 17-year-old me and 72 schoolboys. We stayed in a High School in Munich, which had been turned into a youth dormitory. The army had provided beds and packed breakfasts. It was very well done, and we made the hearty breakfasts last all day. I shared a room with three New Zealanders, one of whom was memorable for her bright green wig.

Initially, the atmosphere at the Games was wonderful. Most days, I picked up my sports bag, and wondered in and out of the Athletes village, where I had friends. Sadly, as history now confirms, security in the village was lax. Then one day, at the school, we were told that the games had been suspended, due to an event, and we were not allowed to leave the school premises. We had no idea why, I think the many young people in the hostel were torn between mild anxiety, annoyance at the disruption and enjoyment of each other's company at the pool.

That night we heard shooting. I now know what was going on was the Munich Massacre; an attack during the 1972 Summer Olympics in Munich, West Germany, on 11 members of the Israeli Olympic team, who were taken hostage and eventually killed, along with a German police officer, by the Palestinian group Black September. We were hearing the failed rescue attempt – at the time we had no idea at all of what was going on. It was quite frightening. I thought we were under fire, and with the curiosity of youth, I crept to the window to see what was happening. We couldn't see anything. Those memories of that tragic night are hearing memories.

I didn't make breakthrough history during my time in Chemical Physics at University; however, I did get a very good grounding in scientific method and in computer science, the main tool of the physicist's trade. With a strong grounding in physical science, it was time to buckle down to sorting out the hearing problems of the world, so I entered a program in Audiological Science, also at Manchester University. The goal of the program was to train physicists to take care of the techy parts of hearing services. It was a model rather like that where radiation physicists work out radiotherapy doses for oncologists. The audiological scientists would take care of the techy bit and audiology technicians and doctors could do the rest.

In audiology, the interwoven worlds of audiology, military action, veteran compensation and hearing aid developments were entering new times. In Britain, we were dominated by the medical model and audiology was really being introduced in order that scientists were available to help the medical professionals. In Britain, if you had hearing difficulties, you were referred by the GP to the Ear, Nose and Throat department of a hospital.

When I started my audiology masters in 1975, I believed I was at the frontier of audiology; the British Society of Audiology was only eight years old. It was started in 1967, with the goal of promoting audiological research, and service quality. At that time, the medical specialty of Ear, Nose and Throat surgeons saw that technology was advancing so fast that greater technical training was needed in the audiology specialty than could be expected from the non-graduate, in-service training of audiology technicians. So the audiological scientist was invented, and I was one of the first.

At that time, post graduate audiology education in Britain was delivered by two key Masters of Science courses, one being through the Medical Faculty at Manchester University, and one being through the Engineering Faculty at Southampton University. The courses were very different in emphasis, but both looked for physics graduates, or something fairly similar. I chose the Manchester course for the simple reason that I was already in Manchester. I had friends there. I liked the athletics track. Why would I leave? I was not very concerned about the difference in emphasis, as I didn't know what was going to be the most important thing to study. I went on in later years to do my PhD in the Engineering faculty at Southampton.

Audiology technicians took an exam managed by the Society of Audiology Technicians & Therapists. I felt a bit uncomfortable when I finished my Masters. I was qualified on paper to be an expert, but with very little practical experience and certainly a lot less than the audiology technicians that I was now senior to. I also realised that our American counterparts had a much more well-rounded professional education. I had some insight into the first post-graduate year, as I was offered a job at Charing Cross Hospital in London, when I had only been on the course for two months. The condition of my early employment was that I worked during the term breaks in my new role as the Audiological Scientist at the new Charing Cross hospital, in Hammersmith. I was to be based in the Medical Physics Department with all the radiation physicists, ten floors away from audiology as I knew it.

My first career role was to develop audiology services of the highest standard, and I was keen to improve my skills and to help generally improve skills in audiology. A logical initiative for me was to become an active, and indeed founder member of a new professional group called the British Association of Audiological Scientists – a collective of people in similar positions to me. As an organisation, we thought that audiological scientists needed more practical experience in their first year of employment, in order to embrace the new role more effectively. In their first year audiological scientists were paid as a provisional scientist (a sort of internship salary), so the NHS authorities agreed that we could arrange a training schedule of practical placements and we introduced an exam to ensure an increased level of professional competence. We called this the Certificate of Audiological Competence (CAC). Structure of the National Health Service, at that time, made this arrangement very do-able. As the NHS was the main employer, it was feasible to train at more than one NHS hospital, in order to get a well rounded experience. It's a model that is not replicable in more fragmented health care systems, such as Australia or the USA. In 1974, an Advisory Committee on Services for Hearing Impaired People (ACSHIP) issued a report that expressed 'deep concern at the extent to which rehabilitation services for the hearing impaired are lacking in the National Health Service'. In response to this, a Certificate in Hearing Therapy was set up in 1978. That is, yet another hearing healthcare professional was invented. This course didn't seek to recruit people with academic qualifications but was aimed at attracting people with some prior experience in working with people with hearing impairment. The graduates of this course formed another professional group called the British Society of Hearing Therapists. The audiological scientist having a senior position in hospitals was often called to be the person carrying out training for both audiology technicians and hearing therapists.

Audiology around the world seems to have developed a confusing and politicised professional landscape. Today, in the UK, there are two registration bodies for Audiologists – the Registration Council for Clinical Physiologists (RCCP) and the Health Professions Council (HPC). Some of the bodies I described earlier, sensibly amalgamated. But alongside the convergence of these professional groups to form a group that would collectively represent audiology, were the medical doctors and physicians. Prominent Otolaryngologist, the late Professor Ron Hinchcliff, who had been my external examiner for my pediatric audiology assessment in Manchester, championed the role of the medically trained audiologist, in the *Audiological Physician*. In 1975, he wrote: *'the audiological physician's role needs to be distinguished also from that of the audiologist. An audiologist is a scientist (or technician). The role and scope of the audiological physician is clarified – audiological physicians are concerned primarily with patients suffering from disorders of auditory communication, equilibrium and spatial disorientation'.*

This last point of Professor Hinchcliff's refers to people experiencing hearing loss and dizziness. Today audiological scientists assess, diagnose and manage patients who have hearing, balance and tinnitus problems. They administer and interpret diagnostic tests to patients. With so many different professionals fighting over our ears, it's no wonder that people are confused.

When I started at Manchester University, I hadn't got much idea of what an audiologist really did. My course was focused on the diagnosis of hearing loss in children, emerging as it had from the history of deaf education. Whatever one's views on oral education, the Ewings had laid a solid foundation in the early diagnosis of hearing loss and intervention. This foundation was put to good use when hearing aids made their oral methods more feasible and acceptable.

As audiology students, we did a lot of work in the audiology clinics, diagnosing hearing loss in babies and children. I loved the clinic work, once I got over my initial nerves. We did quite a lot of our children's clinic work in Pendlebury, which was then the Manchester Children's Hospital. This was in the, relatively brief, time period when medical intervention was getting much better at saving the lives of quite premature and often quite damaged babies, but not so good at fixing them. The hospital had a leading Intensive Care Unit, so there was a concentration of extreme medical emergencies. Even in audiology at Pendlebury, we saw a lot of multiply handicapped children. It was routine to test the hearing of multiply handicapped children, as it is now. However, in practice, there is nothing routine about testing the hearing of very disabled young children. In those days, we didn't have access to the automated detection methods of today. It was all about getting a behavioural response, and it was invaluable experience for a young audiologist.

At the Pendlebury Children's hospital, I was working with children who had chronic conditions that have now become less of a problem as developed countries have become generally healthier. As a student, with limited life experience and no parenting experience, I'm sure I asked the mothers some irritating questions. My total lack of parenting experience and understanding left me inwardly critical of mothers not being able to remember which child had which childhood ailment when. When I became a parent of four children myself, I felt very guilty about those thoughts, because I rarely got that question right. I remember particularly how one mother kept telling me that her child had ear problems, because he was 'different to the other six'. It took me a long time to get to the answer, because I was asking the wrong question. When a mother of seven children says there is something odd about one of her children, then you have to take that very seriously even if you, the smart, new audiologist can't find a problem. I eventually got to the truth, more because of her persistence than any sudden blossoming skill on my part. All her other children had 'runny ears'. This one didn't. This one had perfectly healthy ears, but it wasn't the norm in her family. This was an important lesson for me. I learnt to listen carefully to a parent; ask more open questions; ask to describe what the mother has observed. This also made me think about 'normal'. Normal, used in medicine, education and sociology, is a statistical term, based on measurements in certain populations. At that time, ear health in the industrial north was poor. This mother had seven children and six of them had recurrent middle ear infections. This was so common in her community that it was effectively 'normal' and the infections were left to spontaneously resolve, by the eardrum bursting. Chronic otitis media was normal in her family. I am grateful to my time at Pendlebury and to those wonderful mothers who put up with us students.

At the Department of Audiology, we had an intensive timetable. We would have lectures in the morning and work in a clinic in the afternoon, sometimes in the University Clinic itself, other times in one of the hospitals. It was a rich and fast education and a long way from quantum physics, which is a cerebral activity, enabled by computing. Audiology involves getting information for decision-making from adults and children. You are a lot less in control, and the results are of more immediate need to society.

The method used to test the hearing of little children was that which the Ewings had designed some 30 years earlier, known as the 'The Distraction Test'. The test is still used in hearing screening of young children particularly by maternal and child health professionals. In this test, a child sat on mum's knee, and I would creep to one side and to the back a little, to be just out of the child's line of view. I would gently hiss, or roll the special Manchester Rattle gently. One of my student colleagues would be on the floor in front of the baby, keeping it amused, but being very quiet, distracting the child's attention from me – or, more technically, trying to keep the child's attention to the front. The distracter has to build up a repertoire of interesting, but not too interesting, activities that can keep the child's attention to the front, until the moment that the sound is made, out of vision. The test is suitable for infants with a developmental age of 6–7 months and above. The test is based on the fact that for a child of this age, the normal response to a quiet sound, which occurs out of vision, is a head turn to locate where the sound is coming from. The test works pretty well a lot of the time. The 'Distraction Method' continued to be used in Britain as the principal method of assessing children's hearing well into the late 1970s. Presenting a sound very softly makes a good screening test. The noise makers were chosen to represent both high and low frequency sounds. The staple was the rattle, but it wasn't any old rattle. This was the Manchester High Frequency, or Ewing Rattle. A screening test is a pass/fail situation, where you, hopefully, detect a problem if there is one. In reality, in all screening tests, some problems are missed, and some are falsely identified. The goal is to get the balance between not missing too many children and not over diagnosing too many cases (false positives). That's the essence of a screening test. The Distraction test is used as a screening test of children's hearing in many places today and health visitors and their equivalents in Britain and Australia have used the Ewing rattle for about 60 years.

As students, we had to try and find out how much hearing loss the children attending the hearing clinic had. They were too young for the traditional beep test, but old enough to sit up and react to sound. Tests got progressively more sophisticated as the child got older. More automated methods used today were in early stages of use, but are good to use today, as they can be used over a wider age range.

We learnt to calibrate our voices, and to have a range of sounds, mostly vocal, that we could make at different sound levels until we got a response. Sometimes of course, we didn't get a response. Now imagine me, the slightly hippy audiology student, in a floor length brown corduroy pinafore dress, creeping behind some poor baby and saying 'bub-bub-bub', 'bah' or 'ss-ss' in a very loud voice. When the baby turned its head to the sound, the reward was a grimacing audiology student saying 'Hello' or some such. It must have been bewildering, if not deeply alarming, for both the child and its mother. Periodically, we could check our voice or noisemaker self-calibration with a sound level meter. This test is used today in a more calibrated way, where the sound comes from a calibrated loudspeaker or earphone, and the reward is some kind of animated or illuminated toy. Because it's a bit more interesting, it is used over a wider age range. Although we can now measure hearing responses automatically, there's still a role for what we call behavioural testing – seeing how a child responds to sound.

I have described the 'Distraction Method'. As a child matures he or she becomes too smart for this test, and doesn't spontaneously turn to the sound anymore. Somewhere around 12–18 months the recognition that 'there's a sound back there, and I've heard it before' sets in. Nowadays, this is where Visual Reinforcement Audiometry (VRA), the version with the automated toy, or illuminated puppet can still be used, because it's a bit more interesting than an audiology student off to one side. The age span for VRA is about seven months to about two and a half years. Modern systems use video reinforcement, so that the variety of feedback is much bigger, to keep attention and interest longer. The British were very slow to move to the VRA systems that were in use in the USA, in the mid 1970s, when I was studying. Instead we would carry out a test, rather optimistically known as The Co-operative Response Test, which suitable for children between 18 months and 30 months. I don't know whether this difference was due to NHS economies or was a strong legacy of the Ewings in the teaching of hearing assessment. In the Co-operative Response test, the tester first checks the child's understanding of some simple instructions, and the names of a few objects and toys that you may have laid out. Then an instruction is given at minimal listening levels. If any useful information were extracted from this, some kind of localisation test would be used with high frequency sounds. I didn't ever develop much confidence in this test, though as a screen it had merit. The next stage in developmental hearing tests is like the beep test with training wheels. It's known as 'The Performance Test', is suitable for children between two and five years, and is leading the child towards quantified audiometry. In fact, it's often used as the training or practice run for audiometry. The tester trains the child to perform an action in response to a sound. The ubiquitous toy for this test is a long thin boat with little wooden sailors in it. The child is conditioned to 'put the man in the boat'.

Part of our hearing assessment with children in the two and a half to five year age group, was to also test their hearing with words. We used a test known as The Kendall Toy Test. The Kendall Toy Test, and its derivatives are still being used today to test a child's speech discrimination skills: what I call hearing for speech. The tester sets out a tray of toys, which have been carefully selected so that their names test the child's ability to discriminate between certain sounds. Each toy has a name that fits the pattern, consonant, vowel consonant, known in audiology as CVC words. The child can discriminate between the different words, if he or she can discriminate between the vowel sounds. The vowel sounds are in matched pairs, so that there are pairs of words that sound almost the same. The vowel sounds are the same. The toys have names that are chosen to be easy to confuse. The pairs include: a house and a cow, testing discrimination of consonants in words containing the 'ow' sound; a spoon and a shoe; a fish and a brick; a duck and a cup; a gate and a plate. Then there are some decoy objects too. These are toys that have names that are not part of the pair matching sets. They are just there to make the test more interesting.

The test is particularly useful for children who for some reason are hard to test, for hearing acuity. The Kendall Toy Test, developed by DC Kendall, whilst working with the Ewings, has to some extent been superseded by a more extensive test, called the McCormick Toy Discrimination Test. This version tests hearing for vowels as well as consonants. The author of this test sells a kit of toys, already made up, which is convenient for audiologists. The McCormick Toy Test also comes out of the Manchester audiology stable.

The Kendall Toy Test identifies the child's ability to point correctly to a toy when its name is spoken at a normal voice level. The child isn't allowed to lip read. It relies on clear, controlled diction from the tester. All speech tests are beset with the problem of what to do about regional accents. One of my clinic colleagues had a solution. The tester who is seated in front of the child produces the toys in the test, one at a time, and the child is asked to name each toy to make sure that he or she recognises them, and does actually have a name for them. The tester then trains the child to point to a particular toy when asked a question. I would typically say, 'Show me the...' My Australian clinic partner spent some time asking a child to respond to 'show me the book'. After a few unsuccessful tries she said, 'Show me the book,' (pronounced like the/ oo/ in choose) mimicking a Lancashire accent. The child pointed to the object immediately. Dialect and context affect our hearing. It's harder to both hear and understand when something is unfamiliar. I now didn't need to learn that from a book, however book was pronounced. The same effect occurs when we have to listen to talking when it's noisy. It also taught me not to assume a cultural and linguistic match with the person you are testing. This is becoming more and more of a challenge with word based tests.

The word discrimination tests can identify if a child is able to differentiate between different consonant sounds from within a set of objects. The tests were designed for children whose first language is English, and other tests have been developed to help manage the increasingly diverse linguistic mix that many clinicians are faced with today.

As a student and young adult I had very little to do with small children at all, hearing impaired or otherwise, so I volunteered at a local Government run nursery school to get more 'children practice'. I would collect my two charges, aged two and three, from the large Council housing development flats, known as The Hulme Crescents, to take to the nursery group. The Crescents, as they became known, had more than three thousand flats, accessed from external walk ways, and were organised in crescents as the name described.

My family was on the top floor of one of the crescents: a single mum with three children under four years of age. I don't remember the lift ever working in my weekly visits there over a period of about a year. There was a set of play equipment on the grass within the curve of the crescent. It looked bleak and uninviting, framed on the far side by a new motorway, and was rarely used. I never saw any children there. The secluded stairways smelt of urine; the wind whipped through the crescents in a chilling way, and I was frightened of the dog packs. I thought how pale the children were, which wasn't surprising as they rarely went out. The walls of the flats were thin, so footsteps on the walkway were very intrusive, like the outside world was coming in. This created an odd feeling of being isolated but yet never alone, surrounded, but never safe. There was clearly a lot of vandalism and not much sign of repair. The flat felt damp and cold. I later learnt that they leaked and that few people could afford the under-floor oil fired heating. I hated going there, but I'd been introduced into another side of Manchester life. My impressions weren't unique and the flats were demolished less than 20 years later as a social and architectural failure. At least, thanks to one student, Lisa and Paul got out to playgroup each week, even if my motives were somewhat selfish to start with.

While at Manchester University we did work with adults too, especially in the medical setting. One gentleman I saw had something that looked very strange down his ear – certainly beyond my student experience. I've seen many ear canals and ear conditions now, but this one stood alone and still does. His ear looked very peculiar so I asked him if he had ever had any surgery or medical treatment in the ear. 'No,' he said, 'but I did have a surgical dressing put in the ear during the First World War, when I was in the trenches.' The attending doctor took out the remains of this old dressing, and the poor man found the world offensively and surprisingly loud.

So by the end of the year, I was an audiological scientist, with a Master's Degree and a job in a smart new London hospital. My role was to ensure that all the audiological services in the North West Thames region of England were of a high standard, and that the audiometry technicians were adequately trained for the task. I wasn't, at this point, even too sure what the scope of audiology was. Was I a technician, to fix tricky bits of equipment? Or was I supposed to be crawling round the floor with rattles testing children's hearing? No one seemed to have the answers. I was told it was 'good to be in at the bottom of a new profession', but I wasn't totally comfortable with that degree of uncertainty. Looking back to those days I can certainly see the reason for my confusion. The history of audiology over the last 50 years has been somewhat erratic. I find it hard to define when the study of hearing and hearing measurement became a professional expertise called audiology.

SOME AUDIOLOGY HISTORY

The impetus for the development of the profession of audiology for adults was the Second World War, whilst the impetus around children's audiology emerged more from the education need. The first world course on Audiology was held in 1948, in Stockholm, just three years after the end of the Second World War. During and after the Second World War, there was a need to identify and rehabilitate returning service men that had damaged their hearing as a result of war time service. American scientist, Raymond Carhart became a speech pathologist in the US army Medical Administrative Corps. He was associated for much of his career with North Western University, where he developed rehabilitative audiology. This was at a time when, although hearing aids were not very good, interest in helping people hear and communicate better was rapidly increasing. The Veterans Administration (VA), was established in 1930, and re-organized in 1944. This lead to a big demand for auditory rehabilitation services and both VA clinics and some universities with audiology clinics started to provide government-sponsored aural rehabilitation services for the veterans.

Meanwhile, in Europe, the late Henrik Huizing, of The Netherlands, was one of the first pediatric otolaryngologist and audiologist combinations, and became the founder of the International Society of Audiology. Dr Huizing was one of many at this time writing on the relationship between limited access to hearing and its impact on learning spoken language. He presided, as Secretary of the First International Congress of Audiology, held in Leiden in 1953. Research, education and clinical practice were moving in broadly similar directions around the world, though with different professionals involved. Europe was laying a foundation for an audiology future, where the medical profession was dominant, and where the audiologist would have a strong technical orientation. I was once asked in an audiology job interview in Britain if I could build the equipment, as they hadn't got any. The USA was moving more rapidly to a specialist profession of audiology. Established audiology courses were not driven by physicians and surgeons, and about this time, in 1948, the influential and rightly lauded Marion Downes, of the USA, did her Master's degree in audiology in Colorado. She has helped train generations of audiologists, and I still refer to her famous textbook, *Hearing in Children*, that she co-authored with Jerry Northern. Her status is at least equal to that of the Ewings. She has also been very influential in the establishment of infant hearing screening programs.

One of the several 'fathers' of audiology could be said to be Stanley Smith Stevens (1906–1973), who was based at Harvard University, in the 1940s. Stevens was a pioneering psychologist, who put together a 'Top Team' to study hearing and psychophysics, which was known as the Harvard Psycho-Acoustics laboratory. Among other achievements, Stevens is credited with Stevens' Power Law, which describes the relationship between the magnitude of a physical stimulus and its perceived intensity. The recent history of science is crowded with examples of a thought leader, creating the right environment for progress in their discipline, and Stevens was one of those people. Many psycho-physicists, studying both sound and light, spent impressionable years at Stevens' Lab. His distinguished colleagues went on to include George Miller, whose work we have drawn on with our on-line, scientifically validated Speech Perception test at Blamey Saunders today.

Another alumnus was Hungarian, Georg Von Békésy, who was a pioneer in helping us understand hearing mechanisms, and in testing auditory acuity, but I have always been more interested in how we use our hearing. We need our hearing for spoken communication, if we can't hear words easily, our world is changed. However much theory is written, and however many tests are developed, I always come back to those children in Derby, who were left in no-man's land. George Miller came in to the discipline of psychoacoustics from psychology. He wrote several books and directed the development of WordNet ,an online word-linkage database usable by computer programs. WordNet is an amazing resource it groups English words into sets of synonyms, provides short, general definitions and records the various semantic relations between these synonym sets. He also did a landmark study in 1955, with Patricia Nicely, on 'An Analysis of Perceptual Confusions among some English Consonants'. This is the basis of much work on speech perception research and testing today, including the Blamey Saunders automated Speech Perception Test.

Von Békésy became a Nobel Laureate for his work in physiology and medicine, and he published his first paper on the pattern of vibrations of the inner ear in 1928. During the Second World War, he worked in telecommunications, which made him even more interested in the mechanism and damage mechanism of the inner ear. In 1947, he moved to Harvard University, where he stayed until 1966, when his laboratory unfortunately burnt down.

During his active research career, Von Békésy developed a method for dissecting the inner ear of human cadavers whilst managing to leave the cochlea partly intact, he was the first to show that different sound wave frequencies are dispersed along the basilar membrane in a special way. This happens before the different nerve fibres that lead from the inner ear to the brain are excited. He found that the position of each hair cell along the basilar membrane corresponds to a specific frequency, a bit like keys on a piano keyboard. Von Békésy used his observations to develop a mechanical model of the cochlea, which remained the basis of our knowledge of cochlear mechanics for many years. Through all his years of pioneering research, he had to devise his own techniques and tools. He needed a means to quantify hearing threshold, and so he developed an automated threshold procedure, known today as the Békésy audiometer. This remains as one of the first audiometers.

At a similar time to Von Békésy's studies and foundation work in hearing science, Harvey Fletcher was working at Bell Labs, where he made significant contributions to our knowledge of speech perception. This historic laboratory originated in the late 19th century as the Volta Laboratory and Bureau, founded by Alexander Graham Bell. Bell Labs was also at one time a division of the American Telephone & Telegraph Company (AT&T Corporation), half-owned through its Western Electric manufacturing subsidiary.

Harvey Fletcher showed that speech features are usually spread over a wide frequency range and he developed the articulation index to approximately quantify the quality of a speech channel. He also developed the concepts of equal loudness contours, now commonly known as Fletcher-Munsen curves. These are plots that compare the sensitivity of human hearing to sounds of different pitches.

Hallowell Davis left a huge legacy to audiology and neurology, by developing the electroencephalogram (EEG), and laying the foundation for automated testing that built on the findings of Galvani and Volta. These have become invaluable in measuring hearing in people where some kind of automated method is needed, like babies, or people who for some reason can't cooperate in hearing tests. Hallowell Davis specialised in studying changes caused to the base pattern of the EEG when someone hears a sound. Davis' work led directly to the development of auditory evoked potentials which among other things, allowed diagnosis of hearing loss in infants. It is Hallowell Davis who has been credited with coining the word 'audiology'. He co-authored a book with Richard Silverman, called *Hearing and Deafness*, in 1947 and it remained a key audiology study text for about the next 30 years. The electrophysiology work of Hallowell Davis was continued by Bob Galambos (1914-2010), a neuroscientist who is credited with developing the auditory brainstem response. Galambos was another Harvard man, and performed experiments there, for the military, on the relationship between the shock waves from explosions and hearing loss. He built on the work of Davis, and using electrodes implanted in the brains of animals, he was able to use electronic amplifiers to boost the signals of a single nerve to follow the impulses that travel from the ear to the brain in response to auditory stimuli. This was the foundation of the clinical test used today, the auditory brainstem response, which allowed him to track how neurons respond to the presence of sound at a particular frequency. This research allowed for the development of hearing tests for infants that could be performed by monitoring the brain's response directly to sounds. This is what is now used to complement the distraction tests that I have described already. More pioneering research in human hearing, auditory perception, communication, speech, language and communication disorders emerged from the Harvard Psychoacoustics Laboratories. This included work on sound perception that was important in improving hearing aids and teaching methods for deaf children. Adult speech audiometry was approached in a slightly different way in the United States, to Great Britain, but its American origins were at Harvard. So, the fields started to come together. In Britain, the educators of deaf children were working on better ways to identify hearing loss early, and realising those children needed access to sound to make good use of an oral education method. In the USA, the foundations were being laid after the Second World War, for understanding hearing, and helping people use both hearing aids and their hearing. By the mid 1970s, on one of Britain's first Master of Science level audiology course, I was at the confluence of all this, though I think I wasn't aware of that excitement. Many things are easier to understand with hindsight.

Raymond Carhart became known as the father of the area of audiology associated with learning to communicate better – of rehabilitative audiology. In the same way, Professor James Jerger, another North Western graduate, was the founder of diagnostic audiology, as we know it today – the science of using audiology tests to ascertain the cause of a particular hearing loss. He led the move to establish the American Academy of Audiology at the American Speech and Hearing Association (ASHA) Convention in New Orleans in 1987. This is held as an enormously significant event in the history of audiology in the USA. Today, the American Academy of Audiology, of which I'm an

International Fellow, is the largest audiology member based organization in the world. The establishment of AAA in the USA was clearly an exciting milestone in the history of audiology. I wish I'd been at that meeting.

CHAPTER THREE

WORKING IN TRENDY FULHAM IN THE '70S

When I finished my studies at Manchester University, I had a job to go to, and friends to stay with. I was off to the Charing Cross Hospital in Fulham, London. When I started there, they had a swimming pool that hardly anyone used, and a lot of empty rooms, which there was no money to fill.

I was offered a place on a course called Medicine for Physicists – or how to become an MD in two weeks. It was fantastic. I had a health overview that really helped me understand where my little corner fitted in.

There was a children's audiology clinic, with a well-known medically trained children's audiologist. At least I could confidently help her. Not that she needed much help. There was a big audiology team supporting the Ear, Nose and Throat clinic, managed by an audiology technician, who was an American Masters in Audiology graduate. She had a big team, and certainly knew what she was doing. The clinic evaluated hearing, did tests to find out why people had trouble hearing, and provided hearing aids. These audiology services were all free of course, this was the NHS. It's very logical to have hearing aids provided in the place where hearing loss is diagnosed, and where the cause is investigated. I have always found it odd that in Australia, what public sector hearing aid services there are, exist outside of the hospitals, and I think this has led to the importance of hearing to health being underestimated and marginalised. It makes it hard to integrate the wider health economic impact of hearing loss too. I find today, that it's still hard work to convey to hospitals and health providers in general, the great importance of being sure that people can hear even though we know that hearing loss is under detected in cases of dementia.

Most people will adjust to hearing aids quickly and enjoy a better quality of life if they get on with it early. It's mostly people who leave hearing loss untreated for a long time that need a lot of professional service help to get used to hearing aids. It's very important to get on with using hearing aids as soon as you start finding you have difficulty hearing. Early use of hearing aids potentially avoids significant downstream costs, and it makes economic sense for the individual and for the health system. Researchers, with Dr Frank Lin of John Hopkins University at the forefront, have confirmed that older people with hearing loss experience accelerated cognitive decline, and increased rates of incident dementia. Perhaps more surprisingly, they are also at greater risk of falling. Hearing loss is linked to increased rates of depression, and depression is both tragic and costly. There is also strong evidence that hearing loss decreases ability to self-manage chronic conditions, seek effective treatment, or be reached by public health campaigns. These factors all represent potentially significant health care costs. Hearing loss appears to be associated with lower levels of patient self-management, lower levels of health knowledge, and hence increased health care costs in the long term.

The Deafness, Cognition and Language Research Centre researchers also explain that people with a hearing loss:

'experience greater difficulties in accessing health services, receive a lower standard of healthcare and may avoid going to see their GP because of communication problems. They are more likely to report that they have been left unclear about their condition because

of communication problems with a GP or nurse. Even where patients are able to access health services, hearing loss has a negative impact overall on self-management of long-term conditions.'

These researchers believe that hearing loss may lead to increased rates of smoking, obesity or high blood pressure, resulting in a higher risk of developing some long-term conditions, particularly cardiovascular disease and diabetes. This implies that earlier diagnosis or better management of hearing loss could lower the rate of hospital admissions.

Dr Frank Lin, assistant professor of Otolaryngology, Geriatrics, and Epidemiology at Johns Hopkins University, Baltimore, Maryland, is the principal author of the two main papers demonstrating a link between hearing loss and cognitive decline. Doctor Lin's widely reported study, carried out in 2012, found that a mild hearing loss of 25 dB had an effect on cognitive scores approximately equivalent to seven years of aging, and that in general research shows that cognitive decline and incident dementia are independently associated with hearing loss in older adults. Doctor Lin reviewed the data for 1984 adults, with an average age of 77, who had no diagnosis of dementia. Just over half of the volunteers had hearing loss. He measured their cognitive ability six years later and found that those with hearing loss had a rate of cognitive decline 37% greater than those with no loss and the rate of decline increased significantly with hearing loss. His study showed that hearing aid users did better, but the study has had some critics. Researchers haven't come to an agreement about the cause of this cognitive decline. If a person is socially isolated and withdrawn, this increases the risk factor for cognitive problems. Today people are encouraged to keep socially active, and to remain involved in activities as part of healthy aging. When people can't hear well then they have a tendency to withdraw. Hearing loss due to aging sneaks up; you might say it sneaks up quietly. Age-related hearing loss is a slow, gradual change. It is more marked and there is more impact when there is an existing hearing loss caused by exposure to too much loud sound or noise.

A healthy level of social engagement is associated with a lower risk of dementia, including participating in more social activities, not feeling lonely, and being part of larger social networks. So a common scenario is that hearing deteriorates gradually; it becomes more effort to participate in conversation especially in groups, and the person with hearing loss becomes less and less socially involved. It becomes tiring to participate and less enjoyable as a result. Some scientists think that there is a possibility that the brain may be forced by hearing loss to devote more energy to processing sound, hence losing some of its capacity for memory and thinking.

The ESRC Deafness Cognition and Language Research Centre, based at University College London published a report in 2013 that reads:

'There are good theoretical reasons to support the 'social isolation' theory. The risk of dementia associated with hearing loss appears to increase only at thresholds greater than 25 decibels (dB), the threshold at which hearing loss begins to impact on verbal communication (Lin et al., 2011). Similarly, it has been noted that those people who wear hearing aids do not demonstrate the same level of decline in cognitive function as those who do not (Lin, 2011). Both of these suggest that it is the impact of hearing loss on communication, rather than a biological process, that leads to increased rates of dementia.'

Another significant cost to the health care sector is due to falls. In Australia, 83,800 people aged over 65 attended hospital because of a fall in 2009–10, spending an average of 15.5 days there, according to data published in the Sydney Morning Herald, in 2013. There is a clinically significant association between hearing loss and falls, with a relatively minor loss of only 10 dB enough to see the chance of a fall increase. At a loss of 25 dB, the chance of having a fall reported over the past year increased three-fold.

Dr Frank Lin, has stated that broader health initiatives are needed to inform the public and medical providers about the links between hearing loss, dementia and falls, including early use of hearing aids. Lin says, 'Our findings emphasize just how important it is for physicians to discuss hearing with their patients and to be proactive in addressing any hearing declines over time.' Another researcher at the John Hopkins Medical centre, Dane Genther, MD wrote: 'Policy makers really have to consider hearing loss and its broader health impact, when making decisions, particularly for older people.'

Hearing loss in older adults has been tied to more hospitalisations and both poorer physical and poorer mental health. Organisations exposed to future rises in healthcare costs therefore have cause to consider whether early treatment of hearing loss may be cost effective, in reducing their risk of paying for treatment of other conditions in the long term.

I was in an excellent spot to learn about the importance of planning healthcare services effectively in an integrated manner, and to impact favourably the greatest number of people. My two years at Charing Cross hospital influenced my approach to service provision throughout my career to date. My role at Charing Cross was a bit daunting though given that it was my first career job. My task was to ensure that services in the Health Authority, which I think of as being a fourteenth of the hearing services of Britain, were of a high standard. The North West Thames Health Authority included a lot of hospitals. I was to ensure that services met a high standard and their technical needs were met. My job was to ensure that the regional training centres were up to scratch, and if necessary contributing. I was a new graduate, with very little direct hearing aid experience, and I was in charge. What on earth was I going to do? With a job with such wide geographic responsibility I decided to learn London. Being 23, in London in the 70s was an experience to be appreciated.

After a while I managed to find a flat share in a trendy apartment in Parsons Green, London in 1977. Our landlord, who was an artist, lived on the top two floors of an attractive large Victorian town house. I lived with three other girls on the ground floor and in the basement. There was a pretty little courtyard at the back, hung with plants, making it an oasis in the city. It was Silver Jubilee Year, and much of London was decorated for the whole summer with bunting. London was in party mode.

It was the year Michael Jackson came to London; Fleetwood Mac released Rumours; The Sex Pistols made Punk famous and Frank Zappa, Uriah Heep, Status Quo, Peter Gabriel and Black Sabbath performed just up the road at the Hammersmith Odeon.

We were three girls, who wanted to work hard, establish careers and enjoy London to the full. We were not wealthy, so too poor, a little too far west and perhaps a bit early to be Sloan Rangers, but possibly had the pretensions. Some weekends we opted for country air, and our landlord took us sailing in Hampshire. We exchanged London to wake to the sound of the curlews on the Beaulieu River, as it made its way through the estuary, after its journey through the New Forest.

Sound fills our lives and shapes our experiences and our memories. Today most people in the developed economies should have access to good sound. They don't because of the business models that are allowed to exist. People have been trained to think that they need to spend many thousands of dollars for hearing aids, but they don't. There are now great hearing aids that don't cost many thousands, and I am concerned that there are people in my profession who maintain this practice. In London, the foundations were being laid for a revolutionary company in 30 years' time, but I didn't know that then.

I thought the best way to start my job was to visit all the hospitals in my territory, find out what they did in their audiology departments, what equipment they had, and how it was maintained, happily this turned out to be a good plan. I really wasn't sure how to inspire trust and confidence in people. Why would the hearing technicians be interested in what I had to say? I had swag of degrees, and very little experience. Not for the last time I was very lucky in finding a mentor. I was taken under the wing of the late Professor William Burns, a physiologist who carried out pioneering work on noise damage to hearing. He was famous for his book, *Noise and Man*, and he was based in the Medical school at Charing Cross Hospital. William Burns was one of the first people to understand both how hearing works and what can go wrong. Professor Burns had a laboratory of high quality sound measurement equipment. He was about to retire and had no need for it, so I took it over at his suggestion.

On my travels to the audiology departments in the region, I found that they wanted someone to fix things. I also found a rather inconsistent level of knowledge of the importance of calibrating test equipment. A hearing test compares your hearing to someone else. This only works if the number on the dial produces exactly the same level of sound for every different piece of equipment. Headphones and older style sound measurement systems drifted out of calibration, and had to be periodically reset. This wasn't being done consistently, for several reasons. One was a lack of knowledge of the importance. People would tell me that they didn't have time to get it done, and seemed surprised when I said there wasn't much point in doing the test then. So, happily, inspiration hit. Professor Burns had given me a laboratory of measuring equipment, and so, I should be calibrating the equipment. Happily, the hospital region management supported my idea, they saw that it would achieve a quality improvement goal, and supported my wish to have an electronics technician to help and to fix things. I had possibly sat through a lecture on instrument calibration once. Now, I was alone with the textbooks and the manuals, and it was still 'life before Google'.

Instrument calibration isn't all that straightforward. In audiometry, the pure tone 'beep test', the clinician wants to know how well you hear when hearing is measured through the whole hearing system, from outer ear to brain. This is called measuring hearing by air conduction. The clinician also wants to know how well you hear if the outer part of the ear, the ear canal, and the middle part of the ear is by-passed, causing the inner ear to vibrate, by sending the sound as a vibration rather than as a sound wave. This is achieved by placing a vibrating transducer against the skull, usually, just behind the ear. This is held in place by a springy headband. This would work brilliantly if everyone had exactly the same size head, with exactly the same thickness of skin and bone, but they don't. Not surprisingly, this test, known as the bone conduction audiogram, is less specific than the headphone, or air conduction test. The bone conduction test tests both ears at once, so the clinician has to use quantified noises in the other ear to stop the 'best' ear from doing all the hearing. These test procedures sometimes give the trainee clinician a bit of stress as they try and work out what's going on, or learn 'rules' to minimise the chance of getting it wrong. My current clinic, Blamey Saunders, is also accessible over the Internet, and sometimes people send me their audiograms. I'm sorry to say that I've seen many hearing tests where the air and bone conduction combination have been done incorrectly, or inadequately. My challenge then, was to understand the technical situation well enough to calibrate the equipment. I discovered my ability 'to question' at this point, because I realised that the manuals were oversimplified. There has been some very good basic research done on this measurement technique since then, mostly in Britain.

CHAPTER FOUR

HOW WE HEAR, WHAT CAN GO WRONG AND HOW HEARING CHANGES YOUR BRAIN

'What spectacles are to the eye, the ear trumpet should be to the ear, while the adaptation of glasses to correct the optical defects of the eye, may be considered as one of the complete sciences, with but little more to be desired, the science of Acoustics is still far from furnishing the help required, in the application of its principles to aid defective hearing'
James Campbell, 1882

In this chapter, you are going to read about what an audiological scientist student, in Manchester, might have learnt but with a modern slant, as today's scientific method and instrumentation has given us more knowledge about the ear, hearing and listening. I enjoyed the step from a physical science to an area that encompassed physics, anatomy, physiology and behavioural sciences. It was diverse and needed a breadth of skills. Hearing is a sense, and studying people's behaviour and perceptions is very different to measuring *things,* as you do in physics.

Over the course of my career not only has our understanding of the subatomic world expanded, but our understanding of hearing and listening has changed dramatically. Technical inventions have changed the way we think about hearing and deafness and partially hearing and deaf people have more options than I could have dreamt of in 1976.

Today we can give deaf children access to hearing, from when they are young babies of a few months. Infant screening has taken on much more importance so that no time is lost in giving access to hearing to babies. Many deaf children get cochlear implants when they are very young, and have normal spoken language by the time they are six years old, and then go on to mainstream school. I graduated from audiological science in 1976 and was preparing to work with children and parents who were facing a difficult path ahead – a path that would involve lots of therapy, and where the assistance from technology was inadequate and they would probably never hear. Children were deprived of any kind of language, including sign, because parents and educators were frightened that if a child were taught to sign, they wouldn't learn to speak and would be unable to communicate in the hearing world. Hearing aids now, and even more so then when they really didn't work very well, can only help a hearing impaired person up to a point. There comes a degree of severity of hearing loss that is too severe for a hearing aid to work: enter the cochlear implant. A cochlear implant is a type of hearing aid but, as the name describes, it's surgically implanted. The cochlear implant bypasses much of the hearing mechanism and directly stimulates the hearing nerve bundle.

People don't think much about vision processing when they get glasses, unless like me, they have lots of visual complications. But in some ways many people experience a very quick and easy visual correction, when they don a pair of glasses. Overall, vision is just as complicated as hearing, but the most common reason for mild failures of vision are due to the failure of the lens, and this can be corrected quite easily. It's pretty obvious to the user how the correction is being made. Less common and more severe eye problems are much harder to correct, and research is active in the areas of pharmacology, surgery and the development of a bionic eye.

The most common hearing problems involve distortion to the coding that takes place in the inner part of the ear, so simply making sounds louder, the visual equivalent to lens correction, rarely works. It's harder to fix the common hearing problems with hearing aids, than it is to fix long or short sight with glasses. The cochlear implant bypasses all of this. Hearing aids have got much, much better too. Most of today's hearing aids contain a tiny computer chip, which specialised engineers can program to do sophisticated processing to the incoming and outgoing sound. This is the foundation of my hearing aid company.

The sense of hearing is quite complicated. Lots of people who have lost some of their hearing ability, go to get hearing aids without understanding that getting enough sound in to the inner ear is only part of the solution, and the start of the path to better hearing, better communication and a better life. The full journey takes a little bit of effort, and the longer it's left, the harder it is.

Hearing and listening helps keep the brain fit. People who have very little hearing develop all sorts of brain strategies, using input from other senses. People who slowly lose their hearing, and that's most people, risk losing brain function. The statistics are a bit scary. If you want to get physically fitter, you know you have to exercise. If you want to make the most of your hearing and listening ability, it's not any different. Hearing aids may take a bit of work to get used to and to gain benefit from, and the longer the decision to get hearing aids is put off, the harder it gets because the hearing pathways and the auditory part of the brain lose some of their speech coding functionality, which has to be relearned. Some people are disappointed with even the best hearing aids. This might mean that they have left getting hearing aids for so long that they have really forgotten how to hear and listen or it might be that their expectations are of a miracle cure. The sound through good hearing aids is good but it may not give you access to every sound that you want to hear or block out every sound that you don't want to hear. The hearing aid experience should be a good experience, not a bad experience, but it's imperative to be positive and embrace good hearing and listening habits. It's also important to know that not all hearing aids are equally good, and it's hard for the consumers today to work out how to find good hearing aids. The hearing aid advertisements have been claiming that hearing aids work wonderfully since early in the 20th century. Frankly, at that time, they were not very good. Today many hearing aids are very good.

The hearing process is nothing short of amazing. Every day we hear millions of sounds, and our brain interprets the patterns to make sense of them, and to form judgments on what we need to attend to, and on what we like and dislike. When we hear, we are detecting and coding sound into patterns of electrical impulses. Sound propagation is described within the science of physics, but sound reception, recognition of sound and listening is described within the science of physiology. If a tree falls in a forest, and no one is there, is there a sound? The answer is 'yes' and the answer is 'no' because the word sound is used to describe a physical stimulus, and the word sound is also used to describe a perceptual response. Hearing and listening is truly a case of ear meets brain. Listening is about making sense of the patterns we hear. Listening is also influenced by our personal preferences, our mood, and what we are listening to and even what we are seeing. When we make judgments about the quality of sound or pick out meaningful conversations when lots of people are talking we are not just hearing we are listening. Listening is much harder if the hearing system doesn't work as well as it should, so when it's damaged, hearing aids are used to correct as much of the hearing as possible.

Sound starts as a vibration of an object, and this vibration vibrates the air around, changing the air pressure patterns in a manner that is perceived as having both pitch and loudness. The pressure patterns are usually quite complicated, carrying a lot of information, although we can generate very simple patterns, like the sound of a flute, which is near what we call a pure tone. The pure tone is a very simple wave pattern, where the pressure wave will ultimately move the eardrum back and forth in an even, regular way. If the sound is very loud, then the vibrations and pressure changes are big. The size of the vibrations varies a lot, the pressure wave of the loudest sound the human ear can interpret is 1,000,000 times bigger than the pressure wave of the softest sound it can detect. The sound vibrations might be so big that you can feel them. Scientist Doctor Barry Blesser describes music as a mind-altering stimulant, and says that very loud music is a strong stimulant, which he likens to a double shot of whiskey. He has written a paper with the apt title, 'The seductive (yet destructive) appeal of loud music.' There's a tiny organ in the inner ear, called the saccule, that's linked to the pleasure centres of the brain, and it responds strongly to high intensity, low frequency vibrations. Ear meets brain – again.

A quite different, and perhaps more constructive example, of the body's sensitivity to vibration is provided by the outstanding and famous percussionist, Dame Evelyn Glennie, who is deaf, and uses her sense of vibration to create and enjoy music. She is a versatile and talented woman, who wrote a paper in 1993, in which she describes sound so well that, as a hearing person, I couldn't improve on it. In Evelyn's words:

'Hearing is basically a specialized form of touch. Sound is simply vibrating air that the ear picks up and converts to electrical signals, which are then interpreted by the brain. The sense of hearing is not the only sense that can do this, touch can do this too. If you are

standing by the road and a large truck goes by, do you hear or feel
the vibration? The answer is both. With very low frequency vibration
the ear starts becoming inefficient and the rest of the body's sense of
touch starts to take over. For some reason we tend to make a distinction
between hearing a sound and feeling a vibration, in reality they are
the same thing. It is interesting to note that in the Italian language this
distinction does not exist. The verb "sentire" means to hear and the
same verb in the reflexive form "sentire" which means to feel.'

The pattern of the sound vibration varies a lot. Regular patterns that are repeated over and over are probably musical and most likely classified as musical notes. Musical notes don't need to be made by a known musical instrument, which is why some very strange things have been used as musical instruments, from jam jars to vacuum cleaners. However the sound is generated either by a column of air vibrating or a string of some kind. The grey area of what defines a musical instrument was well demonstrated by the musical humourist, Gerard Hoffnung in his Concerto for Hose-pipe and Strings (Third Movement only) by Mozart, and played in the Festival Hall in London in 1956.

When a sound is generated with a single sine wave frequency component, we call this a pure tone. A key characteristic of a pure tone or a musical sound is that the vibration repeats itself regularly. A non-repeating, random sound is what provides the physical description of noise. There are not many sounds around us that are pure tones. The sound of a flute is near to being a pure tone, depending on the skill of the flautist. Musical sounds that are not noise are usually complex waves where repeating waveforms of the same frequency, but different characteristics are added together. You can think of this a bit like a choir of individual voices being added together.

Generally, if you have a hearing test it is carried out with beep-like sounds, which are pure tones. The microwave beeps are usually nearly pure tones.

Speech is not a pure tone, a pure tone is heard by us as having a certain pitch. However, the vibration of the vocal cords generates speech and the frequency at which they vibrate is known as the fundamental frequency. So for example, many men speak with a fundamental voice frequency of near Middle C or 256 Hz. For most situations, multiples of the fundamental frequency is also heard. These are called harmonics. So for example, if the fundamental frequency is 256 Hz, then the first harmonic is 512 Hz; the second harmonic will be 768 Hz, and so on. A frequency that is double another frequency is, in musical terms, an octave apart. The harmonics give the sound its colour. The harmonics are not heard as separate notes. The harmonics are softer than the fundamental, and when we calibrate, and technically check hearing aids, we are making sure that there isn't an unacceptable presence of harmonic sound. One of the many clever features of the auditory system is that if the fundamental frequency is missing for some reason – let's say it's been filtered out, or is outside the acoustic range of a loud speaker, we still hear the pitch of the note as if it was there. The intervals between the harmonics give us this information. This we may think of as 'The Mystery of the Missing Fundamental'. Ear meets brain.

In speech, the harmonics of speech sounds, specifically, vowel sounds, are called formants. When we speak, the sound is shaped by the opening of the mouth and the position of the tongue, which emphasises some formants, so that the fundamental voice frequency is less important in carrying information. The fundamental is really just setting the voice pitch. Early cochlear implants were designed to use this feature of speech, and to reproduce, in a simple form, the key speech features. The information leading into the formants is important. This is caused by the speech mechanism getting into position. These features are aptly called 'transients' and our brain uses this information in listening to speech.

A really fascinating phenomenon occurs when two tones of close, but different, frequency are presented one to each ear simultaneously. Suppose one ear is presented with a tone at 200 Hz, and the other with a tone of 210 Hz, then the brain hears 10 Hz. This is the phenomenon of binaural beats. When this is done with headphones it's a bit of a trick, artificially recreating a perception that ordinarily would have contributed to localisation. So, if two single-frequency tones are present in the air at the same time, they will interfere with each other and produce a beat frequency equal to the difference between the two frequencies, and known as the difference tone. If tones are presented separately, the same phenomenon occurs.

Some scientists and health professionals attribute mind altering and therapeutic results from attending to binaural beats for a sustained period of time. It's no wonder we are rich with localisation mechanisms. In the past, hearing played a part in the avoidance of being eaten.

The part of the ear we can see is called 'The Outer Ear', anatomically known as the 'Pinna' or 'Auricle', 'Pinna' is Latin for wing or fin. It has a broader role than being a shelf for our glasses. It's a complex shape that is designed to collect sound, and to funnel it in a way that helps us tell the direction that a sound is coming from. The shape of the ear means that it acts as a kind of filter for sounds, and the various shapes and sizes of ears do the job differently.

You are able to localise the direction that a sound comes from, because the sound arrives at your two ears at different times, and at slightly different angles, so the brain does some very fast computing to tell where the sound is coming from, and then can turn attention in the right pinna direction. The pinna is made of complex folds of skin and cartilage and it often gets bigger and floppier as people, particularly men, get older. Big ears are a mixed blessing. They might collect sound better, but children can get very distressed if they have big 'sticky out' ears, even though they can potentially hear better than most people. Big ears can result in teasing, and this can leave the victim feeing unhappy or self-conscious. Today there is a short medical procedure that can reduce the degree to which ears stick out. There is an Ear, Nose and Throat (ENT) consultant called Richard Kang, who was quoted in the Daily Mail in the Britain saying, 'Protruding ears are an aesthetic issue so very much in the eye of the beholder; but up to a million people dislike their ears and improving their appearance can be life-changing. The problem really affects self-confidence.' Despite the efficiency of the pinna, and the potential benefits of big ears, people like neat small ears. The Internet is full of advertisements for ways to pin back ears in young children and babies. Cosmetic procedures mean you can choose the shape of your ears. There are very keen followers of *Lord of the Rings* who get their pinna's changed to 'elfin' ears. The procedure involves cutting off a small wedge of the ear and then stitching the remaining ear to be pointed. The technical term is 'ear pointing'. This will also change their hearing and ability to localise sound. Apparently the procedure is irreversible, so they will go through life with elfin ears.

The path from a generated sound to an interpreted sound starts at the sound source, where a sound wave is generated. Sound waves are ripples in the air, which are really changes in the pressure in the air. The pressure waves are millions of times lower in frequency than electromagnetic radio waves and light waves that can travel through a vacuum. This change in pressure travels down the ear canal, and pumps against the eardrum. Most sounds cause quite complicated ripples. The effect is much like a drumstick beating on a drum, and the faster the vibrations make the drum vibrate, the higher the frequency of the sound. So high-pitched sounds have fast vibrations, and low-pitched sounds have slower vibrations. Similarly, more intense sounds have larger amplitude vibrations than soft sounds.

The pinna surrounds the entrance to the ear canal, which is shaped a bit like a tiny ear trumpet, giving a clue that it might amplify sound, and indeed it does. The pinna and the ear canal, collectively known as the outer ear, collect sound and funnel it down to the eardrum. The sound flows down the ear canal, which is about 2–3 cm long and 7 mm in diameter to the eardrum. The ear canal protects the delicate middle and inner ear. The outer third of the ear canal is supported by cartilage and the inner two-thirds by bone. It bends at the junction of the bone and cartilage in adult ears – that is, about a third of the way down the canal. Children's ear canals are straighter than adults, and the eardrum is more at risk of trauma. The ear canal is lined with a self-cleaning device. It contains a conveyor-belt like system of tiny hairs, lubricated by oily droplets that continuously move dirt and dust to the entrance of the ear canal to prevent the build-up of dust. Earwax, with the medical name of cerumen, is produced by glands in the ear canal, and its function is to protect the ear against foreign invaders, such as microorganisms, dust and chemicals that might hurt the ear canal. After the earwax is produced, it slowly makes its way through the outer ear canal to the opening of the ear. Chewing and talking both help the earwax along, then it either falls out or is removed when you wash. In most people, the outer ear canal makes earwax all the time, but people differ in how much they produce. So you see, earwax is very normal. Wax can be a bit more troublesome when you have something in your ear each day, like earplugs, ear phones or hearing aids, but some simple routines keep it at bay – routines that don't include cotton buds of course. Cotton buds can cause quite a lot of damage because the ear canal is so sensitive, that the roughness of a cotton bud can irritate the skin quite seriously. If your ears produce too much wax and get completely blocked, then it does cause hearing loss. If you have a wax blockage you may experience earache; a feeling of fullness in the ear, a sensation that the ear is plugged, or ringing in the ear. The ear might itch too. Of course these feelings can have other causes. Either way, a trip to the doctor is the best thing to do. Don't go for ear candling though. The theory behind ear candling, which is sometimes called ear coning, is that the heat from the flame will create suction that draws the earwax into the hollow candle, held at the entrance to the ear canal. According to experts at the Mayo Clinic, in the USA, research shows that, not only is it not an effective treatment, but that it can also cause serious injury. Ear candling can lead to deposits of candle wax in the ear canal; burns to the face, hair, scalp, ear canal, eardrum and middle ear and can even puncture the eardrum.

Our ear canal has an acoustic, or hearing benefit, as well as a role in protecting the ear drum. The ear canal is cleverly designed to modify the incoming sound to amplify sounds that are important for hearing speech. The ear and the ear canal are part of the hearing mechanism that conducts the sound to the sensory organ, the cochlea, this part of the ear is aptly called the 'conduction hearing mechanism'. The inner part of the hearing mechanism is called 'the Inner Ear', 'Sense Organ' or 'Sensory Hearing Mechanism', and is where the sound is coded into electrical pulses. The conductive part, which includes parts that you can see, like the pinna and ear canal, has the job of making the sound signal stronger, especially at certain pitches, and introducing information about the direction the sound has come from. The sense organ itself, the cochlea, converts the sound into the electrical impulse that is used by the brain to code sound. The cochlea is named from the Latin for snail shell, which in turn is from the Greek, 'kokhlias' which means 'snail, screw'. Researchers are still trying to understand the full function and mechanism of the cochlea.

The cochlea is filled with fluid, but the conductive part of the ear; the outer and middle parts are filled with air. This is a mismatch that the hearing mechanism overcomes. Water and air have different impedance properties. When sound in air strikes a fluid boundary (a boundary between media with different acoustic impedances) there is a theoretical loss of 99.9% of the energy in a sound wave in air (due to the sound being partially reflected). The air and the fluid have very different densities. You only have to think of trying to hear underwater to know that you can't pick up sound as well in water, as you can in air. The outer parts of the ear make up for this mismatch, by increasing the strength of the sound in the conductive part of the hearing system, just as a transformer allows us to use electrical goods, bought in the USA, in Australia.

The ear canal amplifier is strongest at 3000Hz in the average adult ear. Everyone's ear canal amplifier is a little bit different. It varies depending on their build and the size of the ear canal. Children get more amplification in slightly higher frequencies, and people with ear surgery might get more amplification in the low pitches. Once the ear canal has done its job of making the sound a bit stronger in the mid speech frequencies, the sound wave hits the eardrum. The eardrum is named so because it's a membrane that is like the skin of a drum. Our forebears showed good skills in naming body parts.

The eardrum is a thin, cone-shaped piece of skin, about 10 mm wide. It's quite rigid, but very sensitive, so that very slight air pressure fluctuations will move it back and forth. The ear drum acts like the diaphragm in a microphone or, not surprisingly, like the membrane of a drum. The sound wave pushes the drum in and out. Higher-pitch sound waves move the drum more rapidly than lower-pitch, longer wavelength sounds. Louder sound moves the drum a greater distance than softer sounds.

In this way, the vibration of the eardrum transmits information on the intensity and the frequency of the incoming sound. The eardrum isn't the same thickness all over. The rim is slightly thicker than the rest, and fits into a bony groove in the wall of the ear canal. By this point, the sound is amplified, modified and conveys information about the direction of the sound. The eardrum is the front door to an air filled cavity, which separates the outer ear from the inner ear, once more thus imaginatively known as the 'middle ear'. There are three small bones suspended in the middle ear. The first one, the Malleus, or hammer bone, is attached to the eardrum. This can be seen when someone looks down your ear with a magnifier and light. The bones rock back and forth to the beat of the drum, and are designed to transfer the acoustic energy in the incoming sound for the inner ear.

The middle ear is a bit like a cave with a window made of skin at either end. There is also an escape tunnel from the bottom of the cave that goes to the back of the nose this escape tile is called the Eustachian tube, named for the Italian anatomist, Bartolmeo Eustaci, who described many structures of the human body. Its job is to keep the air pressure in the middle ear at normal air pressure. When the air pressure around you changes very rapidly, such as when you travel in a fast lift, or in a poorly pressurised plane, your ears might suddenly feel blocked. This is because the air pressure in the middle ear has temporarily fallen below atmospheric air pressure. Usually swallowing relieves this feeling, because the act of swallowing helps the air pressure in the middle ear return to normal. The Eustachian tube lets in air, and equalises the pressure either side of the drum. When the Eustachian tube isn't working very effectively, the pressure equalisation may not happen, and ear problems can follow.

The Eustachian tube connects the middle ear cavity to the nasopharynx (the back of the nose), and normally opens and closes periodically keeping the middle ear full of air. When the Eustachian tube isn't working properly and doesn't open and close as it should, then, a negative pressure begins to build in the middle ear space because the mucosal lining of the middle ear absorbs the trapped air. A pressure difference may also be experienced when the Eustachian tube fails to open during ascent or descent in an airplane. Most people have experienced temporary blockage.

This middle ear space has a mucous lining, the body has several cavities that have a mucous lining, and the lining's job is to absorb and secrete fluid, to protect the body against germs. There are also two important muscles in the middle ear, and the facial nerve passes through the middle of the space. This is the nerve that can result in a facial paralysis or Bell's palsy, if it's damaged. The roof of the cave is a thin bone, which is all that separates the middle ear from the brain. This is why it isn't a good idea to leave middle ear infections untreated, lest they cross the divide and cause much worse problems.

The two windows of skin are 'The Eardrum' and 'The Oval Window'. The eardrum is the big main window, and separates the ear canal from the middle ear. The smaller oval window is on the opposite wall and separates the middle ear from the cochlea fluids. The window is the same shape as the stapes, which fits snugly against it.

The difference in the size of these windows plays an important part in the journey of sound to the cochlea. When the sound wave hits the eardrum it is hitting a bigger drum, or membrane, than the oval window membrane. In fact it's generally about fifteen times bigger. Because the vibration from the bigger window is replicated at the much smaller window, by the action of the middle ear bones, the ossicles, the pressure is spread over a much smaller area. In turn this means that it is a stronger force striking the oval window. Think of walking on freshly laid concrete in finely pointed high heels, or working boots. You won't be popular either way, but with the high heels all your weight is focused over a small area, and the heels will make deep holes. The working boots would have spread the weight over a bigger area – bigger footprints but shallower, because the weight has been spread over a bigger area.

This part of the ear amplification is the 'step up transformer' function of the middle ear. It's also part of what is lost with otosclerosis, the condition my dad suffered from. Because the bony overgrowth stopped those bones working correctly my dad started to lose his hearing. Unfortunately when this happened to dad, the problem was not so well understood, and corrective surgery was at a very early stage. In fact when my dad started to lose his hearing he was initially just told by the specialist that, as it was only occurring in one ear, things would be okay. No one would say this today.

The three ossicles or middle ear bones are very distinctive in shape, which is how they got their name: the first bone, the one closest to, and indeed, attached to the eardrum is called the malleus. The malleus, commonly known as 'the hammer', can be seen in a healthy ear, when you look down the ear canal with a suitably focused magnifying light, called an otoscope. I routinely use an otoscope to look down an ear canal to check that the ear canal, and eardrum are healthy and not obstructed by anything that shouldn't be there. Over the years I've seen bits of hearing aids, insect eggs; small toys, beads, hearing aid batteries, seeds and more. The malleus articulates at the top with the incus, commonly known as 'the anvil'. The incus also articulates on the other side with he stapes, or 'stirrup bone', which is the smallest bone in the human body. It rocks back and forth against the oval window, the membrane that separates the middle ear from the inner ear.

My Dad's hearing loss was due to a problem with the ossicles, like Beethoven. When the eardrum vibrates it causes the three little bones to vibrate. They have a big part in making the same signal stronger for transmission into the cochlea. In otosclerosis, unwanted extra bone overgrows the existing bones, starting with the stapes, and stops the rocking and amplification function that the bones would normally perform. If this condition is caught early enough today, surgery can correct it by replacing part of the bone with a tiny prosthetic substitute. Unfortunately though, if it's not caught soon enough, bone grows into the inner ear and causes permanent hearing loss. This is called Cochlear Otosclerosis. This happened to my Dad and probably happened to Beethoven too. The cause of otosclerosis isn't known but it does run in families, and is generally more common in women. Susceptible women usually develop the first signs during pregnancy. Fortunately the condition missed me.

So the sound wave has come down the ear canal, got emphasised a bit to help us hear speech better; has reproduced the vibration pattern on the eardrum, and now the vibration is amplified some more by the middle ear system, and then vibrates the window (oval) to the inner ear or cochlea. Vibration from the eardrum is passed to the malleus first and hence through the other bones, to the oval window. The middle ear is supposed to be filled with air. When your ears feel blocked, it may mean that the air pressure in the middle ear is less than atmospheric pressure, this makes the eardrum less flexible, and means that more sound is reflected, rather than travelling to the inner ear.

The conductive part of the hearing system that we have travelled through delivers the conditioned sound to the inner ear. The inner ear is a very complex piece of coding equipment, with a mechanism that is an evolutionary descendant of some of the earth's earliest creatures of vibration detection – *cilia*. The word, cilia, is Latin for eyelash, and the cilia are hair-like structures that protrude from some cells in the body. Remarkably and perhaps related to this, the inner ear makes its appearance in humans around the 22nd day of embryonic development. The inner ear detects and codes vibrations in the air, by turning the mechanical action of the ear into an electrical representation, the brain does the rest. The ear does this in a way that turned out to be very convenient for the developers of cochlear implants, because the cochlear implant takes the place of the mechanism that turns the vibrations into electrical impulses, and the inner ear is formed so that this happens in a very orderly manner. The inner ear is a bony structure embedded in the temporal bone that's rolled around two and three quarter turns, like a snail shell – hence its name. In fact the cavity contains more than the apparatus, it contains both the cochlear and the vestibular system, known together as the bony labyrinth, and filled with a fluid called perilymph, which is the same make up as cerebral spinal fluid. There are also a series of membranous tubes in the labyrinth, which are filled with a slightly different fluid, called endolymph, which is more like the fluid found in cells in the body. Endolymph and perilymph have similar chemical components, but in quite different ratios, so they are chemically quite different, and the chemical composition is kept in a fine balance. If the composition changes, it can result in hearing or balance disturbances, or both.

The floor of this middle cavity is called the basilar membrane. When the stapes vibrates against the oval window, the membrane sealing the cochlea, it causes the basilar membrane to vibrate. The largest amplitude of vibration takes place at a particular point depending on the frequency of the incoming sound. High frequencies are coded near the base of the cochlea – the nearest part of the basilar membrane to the stapes. The basilar membrane is tuned. Low frequencies are coded near the tip, or apex. In order to make the tip vibrate, the rest of the membrane moves to some degree. This is why low pitches get in the way of hearing high pitches and is one of several reasons why it is hard to hear when there is background noise. There is generally a lot of low frequency energy in noise, and inconveniently, there is a lot of soft high frequency energy in speech. The orderly coding of sound is transmitted through the auditory system to the brain. The sound has to be converted to a neural impulse, and this is done by the hair cell. The hair cell, as the name suggests is a cellular structure on the basilar membrane, that has little hair-like structures on the top, the cilia. When the cilia are bent toward the tallest one in the group, the channels at the base of the cells open and there is an influx of molecules that start the hearing receptor electrical signal. In more biologic terms, we can say that this has caused a neurotransmitter release at the basal end of the hair cell, causing a nerve action potential. The hair cells are not all the same, and can be broadly divided into two types, inner and outer hair cells. There is one row of inner hair cells and three rows of outer hair cells, they both move in response to the travelling wave. The inner hair cells are the primary receptors for sound. Outer hair cells appear to boost the mechanical signal by using electromechanical feedback. The nerve impulses occur most strongly at the point where the basilar membrane has the largest amplitude vibration. The nerve fibres that communicate with the hair cells are also tuned to particular frequencies, the bigger the amplitude, the faster the nerve impulses occur. The frequency of a sound is encoded by the particular fibre that responds, the nerve impulses are passed through various relay stations in the brainstem, and include some crossing over from left to right and vice-verse. The various relay stations in the brain are where some of our senses integrate, for example, the automatic integrations between balance, hearing and vision occur in the brainstem.

The nerve impulses reach the first level of cortical processing at the auditory cortex (the brains hearing centre). The nerve impulses represent the frequency patterns of the sound, and the pattern is replicated in the auditory cortex. This orderly process is called tonotopic organisation, and scientists have found that if an ear has long periods without sound, then this tonotopic representation may become lost. It's one of the many reasons that I try to get people to use two hearing aids, even if the benefit is limited from one. I am not a fan of the CROS and BICROS aids that pick up sound at the bad ear and beam it to the good ear. When I say 'beam' I mean transmit by a wireless method. Previous generations of CROS aids needed a wire to connect the two components. This type of hearing aid picks up sound on one side of the head, and wirelessly transmits it to a device worn on the better ear, so that the sound is routed into the better hearing ear. In my opinion, this is generally the wrong thing to do. Unless the poor ear has no hearing at all, it is better to keep it active for as long as possible, and to provide amplified sound so that it is kept active. Hearing is a 'use it or lose it' sense, so we need to let both ears 'use it' if possible. One hemisphere tends to be more important than the other for a wide range of auditory stimuli and experience. Processing of speech is localised to the left cerebral hemisphere. Music is more right brain, having a strong emotional emphasis.

The brain has to make sense of the patterns that are delivered. Imagine that you are looking at a musical score. There is a melody there and at any one time there are multiple notes being played perhaps by a piano or perhaps by multiple instruments. Your ear codes all the different components and then at the cortical level you hear a melody with a certain texture depending on the components at any one time. If you are an orchestral conductor you can probably tune in to the components but most of us don't. We can think of speech in the same way. We have the ability to pick out information in quite complex auditory scenes, even though the sound in the auditory scene all come together to make the same signal that enters your ear. It is at the level of the brain that we work out the correct sound. That's why it's important when you get hearing aids to keep using them so that your brain has a chance to re-learn how to interpret the auditory scene.

CHAPTER FIVE

How well can you hear?

The most common method for measuring hearing sensitivity is pure-tone audiometry, which is carried out at frequencies of 250Hz to 8000 Hz, in octave intervals, for no particularly good reason. The manufacturer of the first audiometer chose this pattern, and it seems to have been since enshrined into some sort of audiological fundamental truth. The method of pure tone evaluates the whole hearing pathway from the external ear to the auditory cortex. In other words, a beep is presented, processed by the ear, transmitted to the brain, recognised, and the listener then indicates by some action, that they have heard it.

BEEPS, WORDS AND COMPENSATION

I am not a fan of the 'beep test', commonly used as a hearing test. The 'beep test', has become a traditional way to measure hearing, since the first audiometer was produced by – guess who – Western Electric, that relation of Bell Labs. Indeed, the invention should probably be attributed to Alexander Graham Bell. Western Electric produced only about 25 of these audiometers, which retailed for $1,500 in 1923. This cabinet sized unit had sliding glass doors over the controls. Below the controls was a shelf protected by leaded glass and a curtain, with a wooden storage drawer at the very bottom. In this audiometer, vacuum tubes served as the sound source and amplifiers.

The audiometer is used to measure the softest sound you can here at a range of frequencies an octave apart, chosen by the Western Electric engineers. Carl Seashore introduced the audiometer as an instrument to measure the 'keenness of hearing' whether in the laboratory, schoolroom, or office of the psychologist or 'aurist'. Seashore's audiometer was not the first attempt to create an instrument for hearing testing; however its ability to attenuate intensity logarithmically made it a landmark invention. The Council on Physical Therapy of the American Medical Association organised the first attempt at standardisation by releasing tentative findings in 1937. It was not until 1951 that the American Standards Association (ASA) introduced audiometric zero based on normative values.

The audiogram is measured using an audiometer, which presents tones of different frequencies to the client through calibrated headphones, at specified levels. The levels of the tones at the different frequencies are weighted to a standard graph known as the minimum audibility curve. This is a measure of threshold at different frequencies, obtained from a cohort of healthy young people. The resulting mean is used to represent 'normal' hearing. The weighting is necessary as the human ear is not equally sensitive to sounds over the range of frequencies. There are several versions of the minimal audibility curve, defined in different international standards. The ASA 1951 standard, for example, used a level of 16.5 dB SPL (sound pressure level) at 1 kHz, whereas the later ANSI-1969/ISO-1963 standard uses 6.5 dB SPL. A 10 dB correction is allowed for older people. In pure tone audiometry, tones are presented at specific frequencies (pitches) and intensities (loudness levels). The client indicates when he hears the sound. The lowest intensity heard at any one frequency is recorded as the threshold. The result is a map of hearing acuity to pure tones, at different frequencies, with no competing background noise.

This graph, the audiogram compares your hearing to someone else doing the same beep test, and if you have it done at different periods of time, it tells you how your results have changed, but other than that it's not a very informative test. It's confusing to the person being tested, causes unnecessary anxiety, and doesn't actually give very useful information.

The audiogram measures at what sound level you can hear 'flute-like' pure tones, in a very quiet room. Audiology has become rather traditionally dependent on the audiogram, and it has become widely accepted, despite its shortcomings. How did this happen? Like many things in science and medicine and commerce – it's come about by a combination of events, but spread over such a long period of time that people seem to have forgotten why. No learned body ever met, deliberated and decided that the audiogram was the best path or method to establishing hearing difficulty, although there have been many studies showing the degree of correlation, on average, to hearing difficulty.

The term audiometer, and the professionals who use them, have an interwoven history. Use of the terms 'Audiology' and 'Audiologist' in publications only date back to the 1940s. Remember Stanley Smith Stevens, the psychologist, who pioneered psychophysics, at the Harvard Psycho-Acoustics laboratory? His Nobel Laureate colleague, Békésy, published his first paper on the pattern of vibrations of the inner ear in 1928, and developed an automated procedure for measuring hearing thresholds, known today as the Békésy audiometer, about the same time.

Professor James Jerger, played a major part in integrating the audiogram into diagnostic audiology. If the audiogram is carried out using headphones that carry the sound, what is known as air conduction that is, as an acoustic sound wave to the eardrum, and is also measured by a calibrated vibrating transducer commonly known as a bone conductor, then it is possible to quantify how much of a hearing loss is due to the conductive component of hearing that is, the middle ear mechanism.

There have been other methods to determine hearing ability, before and since the invention of the first audiometer. One of the proposed methods for early diagnosis of hearing loss includes measurement above the original boundary test frequency of 8kHz, now known as extended high frequency audiometer. I worked on this area as part of my PhD, as commercial systems were not available at that time. Exposure to noise affects our hearing for high frequencies sooner than conventional frequencies. By the time you can afford an extended frequency response Hi-Fi system, there's probably not much point in buying one.

There are new, sensitive and automatic ways now to measure early hearing deterioration, which uses an interesting curiosity of our hearing mechanism. We can measure something called the oto-acoustic emissions from the ear. This is the measure of the energy that is made by the inner ear, in other words, it's the noise the ear makes when it hears. Even slight hearing damage can be detected by measuring the sound of hearing. It doesn't tell the tester how well you can hear, and use sound, it is an automatic test of the hearing function.

Noise induced hearing loss, known as NIHL, is among the most common occupational diseases. Workers exposed to noise are regularly evaluated by conventional audiometry to find cases of NIHL, an irreversible disease. It's hard to force workers to protect their hearing, so hearing protection is not universally used. Early diagnosis of NIHL or early detection of ears susceptible to the effects of noise can prevent hearing loss from getting worse and involving the sound frequencies that are important for hearing speech. Researchers have found that the frequencies of 4000, 6000, 10,000, 14000 and 16000 Hz are the frequencies that are affected first by loud sounds. A hearing conservation program is one in which a community or an employer seeks to help protect people's hearing. Hearing is usually monitored, and the participants are encouraged to use hearing protection or avoid the loud sound levels. A hearing conservation programme will generally include some kind of hearing monitoring. Most commonly, this is just the standard audiogram, but, as we've read, better methods are the use of either oto-acoustic emissions or high frequency audiometry.

I much prefer the idea of someone acknowledging their own hearing loss than having someone tell them by a beep test. This doesn't work for paying compensation or quantified monitoring, but it works very well as a measure of difficulty. The next best thing is to listen to words, in a manner that tells you what sounds of speech you can hear, and which you can't. That's why we invented a new test. It's time to move on from the days of the original Western Electric Audiometer. Using speech sounds to test hearing is not new. The step we took was to make it self-administered, and to provide an analysis that's meaningful. We call this The Infogram™.

The audiogram is commonly the first test, and sometimes is the only test, carried out at an audiologist's office, clinic or hearing aid centre. This varies from country to country. The audiogram, though, commonly under-estimates hearing difficulty. It's not uncommon to hear someone who is having hearing difficulties emerge from a hearing test to triumphantly say they've passed. My husband John did this. I wasn't having that and got hearing aids on him. He's very happy with them, but disappointed that car engines hadn't improved in acoustic properties as he had thought before he got hearing aids. Sticking to an audiogram made sense years ago, but it doesn't now that hearing aids are better. Getting a 'Pass' on an audiogram, when you have hearing difficulties that could be corrected is just going to make life harder, later. The audiogram is a numerical measure of the sensitivity of hearing that has been in use for the last 100 years, since the invention of the audiometer.

The ability to discriminate between sounds of different frequency is a important part of speech recognition. Discriminating between different frequencies is substantially what we do when we discriminate between different speech sounds. Frequency selectivity is the ability of the normal ear to tune in to narrow frequency bands. The pure tone audiogram does not measure this aspect of hearing.

I have observed that people like 'a test' to confirm a problem. It's as though we need someone else to validate our experience, but the audiogram is not 'the right test'. If the audiogram doesn't give answers that explain the problem, and frequently it won't, that doesn't mean you or your family are imagining the problem. The conventional screening audiogram does not pick up mild hearing difficulties that can be sufficient to cause considerable communication difficulties and changes to lifestyle. The test is not even particularly good as a tool for setting up hearing aids. It is actually quite inconvenient to have a measure where the actual pressure levels that vary across the frequency range according to the variation in 'average normal hearing', as a result of using a weighted approach to tone presentation at different frequencies. Scientists have almost made an industry of developing formulae to try and set up hearing aids from audiograms. It's one of the reasons that hearing aids have traditionally needed an expert to help you set up.

It turns out that the time gap between people developing hearing difficulties and seeking help is remarkably long, typically 7–10 years. There are lots of reasons for this, but it includes not taking the early signs of hearing loss seriously, and not realising the great importance of getting on with using hearing aids sooner rather than later. Several large research studies have re-iterated the importance of taking note of your own, or your friends, observations that you are not hearing, so if more confirmation is needed, then that's the real test – not the beep test. I realised that a test was needed that gave people the confirmation that they weren't imagining their difficulties, and that gave a bit more information about their hearing. We also wanted something that was easy for people to find and do, so we made it free and put it on the Internet. No need to wait for your turn on the waiting list. No need to go out. No need to face people trying to sell you hearing aids. So we developed and launched the Blamey Saunders SPT® (the acronym for Speech Perception Test). Speech tests always seem to be named after their inventors, or after a local river. I guess it could have been the 'Yarra SPT'.

It has been known for some time that speech recognition tasks of one type or another are important in the assessment of hearing ability. As long ago as 1976, Reinier Plomp, a well-known hearing scientist writing in a time of less sophisticated hearing aid technology than we have today, wrote about weaknesses in speech recognition that people with hearing impairments experience, involving both a softening, or attenuation and a distortion of the acoustic signal. Attenuation of the acoustic signal is directly shown when the thresholds measured by the audiogram are raised. The pure tone audiogram demonstrates that low amplitude portions of the speech signal will be inaudible, that is, the softer parts of speech will be inaudible. Although word tests have been used before in general audiological practice, there has never been a freely available test that gives a detailed breakdown of the speech sounds that you can hear, and the ones that you don't hear. Word tests have more commonly been used in the past to evaluate the usable range of hearing or to confirm audiometric thresholds, and there is still a place for these tests in clinical practice, just like there is still a role for the audiogram in finding out what part of the hearing mechanism is causing the hearing loss. The Blamey Saunders SPT builds on previous research and clinical experience.

It's also useful to use words to see how well your hearing aids are helping you. People use this test at home to see how well they can hear with their hearing aids on. Understanding speech involves the brain, so testing hearing with speech sounds is a more realistic picture of how someone really copes.

Gary Lawson and Mary Peterson have written a book called simply *Speech Audiometry*, which is intended for audiology students. In their book, they wrote:

'While pure tone audiometry by air and bone conduction provides good information regarding the basic types of hearing loss, it provides limited and indirect information about how we hear speech. Speech audiometry can tell us how well one hears speech.'

An advantage of the Blamey Saunders Speech Perception Test is that the listener sets the speech at a level they find comfortable to listen to, which is usually the sound level where they hear the best, so the test is sort of self-calibrating. Ken Grant of the Walter Reed National Military Medical Centre wrote a guest editorial in the 'Journal of the American Academy of Audiology' in April 2013.

'From the beginnings of audiology the focus has been to compensate for loss of audibility. However we all know that there is far more to the story for the typical clinical patient presentation of "I can hear. I just can't understand". Compensating for loss of audibility is the low hanging fruit in signal processing for impaired hearing.'

Speech sounds, presented at real world levels give us more insight. It also means that the clinician doesn't have the sight of an anxious client, holding their breath, in order to try and hear the softest sound. It means that you are not setting pure tones at a threshold in competition with the client's own tinnitus.

The normal data for the Blamey Saunders SPT was collected from individuals who did not report any hearing difficulties and were considered to have good otological health. Although it correlates well with the pure tone audiogram, that is almost irrelevant. The test is a substitute, and the correct comparison is difficulty, not pure tone audiometry.

Speech in noise tests are useful for quantifying how much trouble someone has in understanding speech in background noise. I like to use this test with my clients, in my office, or clinic with the client not wearing hearing aids, and then wearing them, to see if the hearing aids are effective. Good hearing aids will help, by making the level of the speech that reaches the ears, louder in relation to the noise. This is called, improving the signal to noise ratio. A number of clinicians and researchers have said or written of the inadequacies and limitations of the audiogram, but there have been few attempts to find something better. The pure tone audiogram does not identify frequency selectivity and temporal frame structure. Scientists agree that performance on these tasks is correlated with speech recognition performance, however accurate modelling of the details is as yet incomplete.

In a recent interview with the American Academy of Audiology (Web Watch 2014 American Academy of Audiology), Professor Jay Hall, Author of the student text, *Introduction to Audiology Today*, says:

'The audiogram was never intended to serve as the basis of counselling and it was certainly never meant to be the basis of a hearing aid fitting. Yet, it's used every day, in most clinics around the world, for exactly those purposes. And so, as I said in the book, the audiogram is undoubtedly very valuable, but it's not a true or comprehensive test of hearing. That is, we hear with our brains! The audiogram just measures a small fraction of the frequencies we might perceive, and it's just a measure of detection, not comprehension or recognition, and the patients don't listen to pure tones in the real world, they listen to words in noise, and so I totally agree with your core premise. The diagnostic battery needs to be recognized as just that, and then we need to perform other pragmatic, scientific and audiologic protocols to address the patient's listening problems, many of which have a cognitive or processing or perhaps other basis.'

CHAPTER SIX

THE SOUND OF TREES, THE NOISE OF TRAINS

I wonder about the trees.

Why do we wish to bear

Forever the noise of these

More than another noise

So close to our dwelling place?

-

Robert Frost, The Sound of Trees

Hearing and listening is a complicated mix of physical detection, neural coding, subjective perception and even emotion. We might think of hearing as detection, and more sophisticated processing as being part of listening. But of course they are fiercely interwoven. We might think of listening as 'where ear meets brain'. So let's leave the story of the measurement of hearing for a while to think about listening.

Spoken language and music perception are the strongest examples of where ear meets brain. Knowledge of sound and sound measurement is important to control the physical stimulus, for sound production, hearing aids, telephony and many other purposes. Our ears measure pressure differences not loudness and our ears are both very sensitive and able to operate over a very wide range of pressure differences. The auditory system is so sensitive that it can detect pressure changes that at the eardrum cause less movement than the diameter of a hydrogen atom. If hearing was much more sensitive we would be able to hear air molecules colliding. Yet the pressure difference between the sound of soft rain and the sound of a chainsaw is about a trillion times. Measuring sound in a way that makes sense to talk about has resulted in the use of the decibels, which is a ratio of two physical measurements of pressure. The sound pressure of a sound that we would find painfully loud is about a million times greater in sound pressure than the softest sound we can hear; 20 million micro μPa vs 20μPa. This doesn't make a very convenient way to measure sound, partly because the softest sound is not zero Pa (pressure units). Thus the decibel scale, which is a ratio scale, was invented, where the softest sound that an average group of volunteers could hear was established as 0 dB SPL (Sound Pressure Level).

The perception of loudness is the reality of the sound in the mind of the perceiver. Everyone is different. That's why to me it makes no sense at all to fit hearing aids to predictions, based on averages. Loudness is the subjective perceived auditory sensation, which arises as the result of the strength or amplitude of a sound. Increasing the sound pressure of a tone increases its loudness. We measure loudness in units called the sone. The loudness of the sound depends on its frequency as well so we can't tell how loud a sound is just by saying the sound pressure. We have to quote the frequency of the sound as well, because the human ear is more sensitive to some frequencies than others. In other words we don't judge sounds of the same sound pressure level, but at different frequencies to be equally loud. People with normal hearing are most sensitive to sounds around 2–4 kHz, and less sensitive either side of this zone. Children can hear up to about 20 kHz, although they are much less sensitive to the very high frequencies than around the 2–4kHz. Sensitivity to high frequencies deteriorates over our life for most people. By the age of 55, perception of sounds above 4kHz is commonly much reduced, and by 65 sounds above 2kHz need much higher input. Sadly, these sounds that need increased levels to hear are also important for hearing speech sounds.

Because our ears respond to pressure changes, scientists have developed a measurement system that relates to the measurement of pressure, but it was devised in a roundabout way. The result is that the numerical relationships may not seem very obvious at first. Doubling the sound pressure level gives an increase of 6dB. If the sound pressure is ten times as much, the sound pressure level is +20dB. Put the other way around, when we increase the sound pressure by a factor of ten, which is the same as increasing the DB SPL by 20 this ear increases the loudness by a factor of about four.

I said 'about' four, because loudness is a subjective feeling and is a little bit different for every individual. So, perceived loudness of a sound depends on several factors: the amplitude, the sound pressure level, the frequency, and also the time behaviour of the sound. It even depends on other simultaneous sensory experiences.

The effect of duration on loudness is still the subject of scientific study. It is generally found that for a given intensity, loudness increases with duration up to 100–200ms. Once that plateau duration is reached, the loudness is not affected by further increases in duration of the sound, although there are some differences depending on the intensity of the sound.

The loudness of a sound is affected by the width of the frequency spectrum that is involved in the sound generation. We call this the 'bandwidth' and the wider the bandwidth the more detectors in the inner ear are involved. Generally speaking, and it is of course a bit more complicated than this, if more detectors are involved, then a sound is perceived as louder.

Our perception of loudness is affected to a surprising degree to what we are seeing at the same time. For example if we see a single flash of light at the same time as we hear a series of beeps we have the impression that the light is flickering. If a disc is flashed once and is accompanied by one to three beeps, then we perceive it as having flashed twice, the extra-perceived flash is illusory. By changing the pattern of beeps, we can increase or decrease the number of flashes that we see. It used to be thought that vision was entirely dominant over our auditory experience, but more recent research has shown that it is sometimes the other way around and our auditory sense can alter our visual perception. Researchers have shown that sound is the more dominant sense when timing is involved, and vision is more dominant when a sense of space or location is involved. This is because the ear codes the timing of sound more finely than the eye, and the eye is better at coding spatial information than the ear.

We can discriminate between single and pairs of click sounds when they are separated by a gap which is only a few tens of microseconds long, whereas it's hard to see the flicker of a light unless the gap is about 2000th of a second. A great example of visual dominance, due to a location effect, is the ventriloquism illusion. Ventriloquist entertainers became popular in the 18th century and have understood for a long time the entertainment value of confusing perception with a mixture of vision and audition. You may see a ventriloquist's dummy's lips moving, but you hear the sound coming from the ventriloquist. It's an audiovisual trick, with vision dominating. According to your auditory system, the sound seems to be coming from the ventriloquist's mouth, but your brain picks the visual cue – the ventriloquist's dummy.

It is disturbing if the audio and the visual are not synchronised when you watch a film. Perfect synchrony isn't always possible due to technical constraints. The human brain is accustomed to a certain amount of asynchrony between auditory and visual information due to the fact that sound travels more slowly than light, but if it's too much, then it becomes an adverse and distracting effect, and the effect is also slightly worse if the visual clip is leading rather than lagging. Researchers have sought to find out how mismatched audio and visual have to be for us to detect it. We have the lowest tolerance for time difference between simple non-speech sounds, higher for speech, and highest for piano and guitar music.

Our hearing and visual processing for speech are somewhat interdependent, and our ability to use hearing and lip reading together is consolidated by the time we are about six months old, and we can identify what a person is saying when there is background noise, better if we can also see the speech clearly. If you need glasses, you will hear better with your glasses on. The hearing part of the brain even has a special component for this interesting phenomenon. There is a region in the auditory cortex in the brain that is used for audiovisual processing of speech.

Although the auditory system is not as accurate, or dominant in location as the visual system, hearing a sound acts as an alert or warning for the eye to turn to an event that was previously out of view. This is exactly the mechanism being used in the children's hearing test, the distraction test. When a sound and a light are perceived at the same time, observers respond to the stimuli more quickly than they would to either of the stimuli alone.

We refer to the perceived intensity of sound as loudness and to the perceived intensity of light as brightness. Both loudness and brightness depend on the characteristics of the specific stimulus, sound or light and on the context in which the stimulus appears. The intensity, or loudness, of a sound can be used to convey the importance or urgency of a signal. The ear, or hearing, has a role in alerting us to stimuli. In fact hearing interacts with other parts of the brain so that a warning signal will produce an immediate general reaction leading to escape, a quickening of the heart rate, a tensing of the muscle and a readiness to move. Hearing links in to the body's fight or flight response, which is a throwback to our caveman days. Unsurprisingly, loudness of sounds is related to how annoying we find the sound, but perhaps surprisingly, both the size and the colour of some objects affect our perception of loudness, and hence, probably annoyance. This interaction of sound and colour works the other way round too, so that the sensitivity to a green light increases as an accompanying sound intensity is increased, and the sensitivity to an orange-red light decreases as the sound intensity is increased.

There was a researcher who showed that red sports cars sound louder than other coloured sports cars. Dark green follows a close second, but pale green is not so loud. This experimenter showed pictures of a sports car in different colours to his volunteer subjects. The dark-green colour was digitally modified, so that in addition to the original colour, the images of a red, blue, and light-green car were shown to the volunteers. The participants in the study listened, through headphones, to a recording of an accelerating sports car that lasted for a few seconds. The participants had to rate the loudness of the sound each time, and the researchers found that they judged the loudness differently, depending on the colour of the car in the picture. The influences in this study may not be well understood yet. We know that a combination of colour and sound can raise physiological excitement and that a feeling of excitement may contribute to actually over-estimating loudness, so the influence of the expectation around red and dark green can't be eliminated. There are also whole books in psychology devoted to the interaction of colour on mood and arousal that show what an involved and interesting field of study this is. One researcher in a big hearing aid company once told me that they had more hearing aids returned, because the user didn't like the sound, if they were red, than any other colour hearing aid, so they stopped making red hearing aids.

The Ancient Greeks were probably the first people to have made a scale of musical notes that were linked with colour. This was based in Aristotle's theory of colour, which was considered valid into the 17th century. Different colours were associated with various tonal intervals in the 17th century.

There are some people who have a special synergy of the senses. In fact it goes further than just synergy. When one sensory or cognitive pathway leads to automatic and involuntary experiences in a second sensory or cognitive pathway, it is known as synaesthesia. The experience is as though their senses are joined. There are people who see colour when they hear sound, or vice versa, although these are not the only percepts that can be affected.

The composer Franz Liszt was thought to have synaesthesia, and an anonymous quote was recorded in a book by Friedrich Mahlingin in 1926:

'When Liszt first began as Kapellmeister in Weimar in 1842, it astonished the orchestra that, he said: "O please, gentlemen, a little bluer, if you please! This tone type requires it!" Or: "That is a deep violet, please, depend on it! Not so rose!" First the orchestra believed Liszt just joked; more later they got accustomed to the fact that the great musician seemed to see colours there, where there were only tones.'

Musician and performer Kanye West has been very public about his synaesthesia, and said in an excerpt from an interview with Seth Meyers on *Late Night with Seth Meyers*: 'I have synaesthesia. I can see sounds in front of me.' Apparently, for Kanye, pianos are blue, snares are white, and bass lines are dark brown and purple. It seems that Kanye West is part of a growing number of elite artists coming out with their synesthesia.

The interaction of loudness and colour is now sometimes investigated in order to work out whether a particular product will be annoying. One study on the effect visual cues have on loudness judgement showed that people rated a noise louder when seeing a picture of a big truck, than when they saw a picture of a small truck. This seems to lead to the possibility of offsetting the annoying loudness of large trucks by spraying them pale green. But how do we actually decide what is noise? Is all background sound noise, because it stops us hearing so well? What about music in a supermarket? Is that noise or is it relaxing.

Noise is another subjective phenomenon and the hearing aid manufacturers both nightmare and opportunity. And thinking of nightmares, look at how noise is used in Gothic horror stories: howling wind, doors squeaking or slamming shut, sighs, moans, howls, sounds of footsteps, clanking chains, dogs howling or unusual laughter. If noise can be used so easily to create an atmosphere of fear, perhaps it's logical that the word, noise, probably comes from the Latin *noxia*, meaning 'harmful things'. The hearing aid manufacturer's nightmare is different. The challenge for a hearing aid is to differentiate from sound you want to hear and sound you regard as noise. It's technically much easier when you are working in the area of Bluetooth headsets or telephony for the engineers to decide that noise is anything other than the conversation between two people. That's presumably why you are using the phone – to talk to someone, and you want it to be as easy as possible. When I was running the company Dynamic Hearing, the CEO of one of the companies that we were working with said he wanted a noise cancelling solution that was so good that he would be able to use his headset, when standing beside a tram.

But what if you are not designing telephones? What is noise then? We have all heard of the difficulty of hearing when a lot of people are speaking in a room. This has the rather dated name of the 'cocktail party' effect. Undoubtedly this is a hearing and listening challenge for people both with and without hearing aids. If you are using hearing aids, with microphones that are directional in that situation, and you have the discipline to turn your head to the person speaking and you are not far away from that person, then you will get quite a lot of benefit from your hearing aids. I rather shamefacedly admit that I don't do as I advise and I don't wear my hearing aids all the time. However, I always wear them when I am in a situation where a lot of other people will be talking. My hearing aids are our own Blamey Saunders hearing aids and have adaptive directional microphones that work in this situation. So let's assume that we are at an event where lots of people are talking. Lots of people are talking, in a big room, and sound is being reflected off the walls. The multiple sound reflections off the walls mean that the same original sound can reach the ears several times, but at different times and from different directions. This effect is known as reverberation. All in all, it's a tricky listening situation, even if you have really good hearing, but it's a tough spot for hearing aid users. Getting around that particular listening problem is technically complicated. We could cut out all the background noise. But the noise is mostly speech, which we probably don't want to cut out, although one client of ours suggested that we should find a way that her husband's hearing aid should only be able to pick up her voice, and that everything else could be treated as noise. Let's suppose that there's a very interesting looking person in a gorgeous jacket, looking very animated, but not directly close to me. Suppose this is a person that I want to overhear. Our hearing aids are designed to make sounds audible and comfortable, but not to choose particular sounds for people to hear. My philosophy is that hearing aids should make the signal as clear and intelligible as possible and leaves the brain to do the rest. The hearing aid is unlikely to know that I want to overhear the bloke in the gorgeous jacket. In this situation, we do need to use all our hearing and listening skills, including attention, memory, and our ability to know where sound is coming from – what is called, spatial processing.

It is still not fully understood why people have so much difficulty hearing in background noise. Background noise will certainly test your hearing aids and some will perform better than others but it is also how you use them. When I am working as an audiologist in my hearing clinic, I do a lot of testing of hearing against background noise. Because people are so variable in ability,

I use a range of different measurements, this helps me to advise people how to manage their hearing. If you are getting hearing aids and you are choosing to do it through a hearing clinic then it's a good idea to ask if you can have these assessments done. In the cocktail party type situation hearing aids are certainly not a miracle fix, but remember that everyone has difficulty in this situation. Draw on your other skills, and encourage other people to do the same. When people find sounds annoying, and the sound is persistent, they can get side effects, which include increased heart rate and increased blood pressure which, among others, may lead to hypertension. This is the reason that so much attention is given to airport noise, and wind farm turbine noise.

Whether something is noise or not depends on other factors, such as its perceived loudness, pitch, continuity, variation with time, time of occurrence, cause or origin and the recipient's state of mind and temperament. I once lived opposite a railway junction, and the bedrooms in the house faced the rails. The sound of the trains didn't keep me awake at night, but my visitors usually found it hard to rest. I was used to the sound, but I also quite liked it. However, many years later, when I lived in an apartment in an inner city area, I hated the sound of the squeaking garage roller doors and the repeated nocturnal crashing of the garbage trucks which seemed to be frequent. I found it hard to sleep. I disliked what I termed annoying noise. Where I live now out in the country, the frogs in the pond are probably just as loud as the garbage trucks, but I love that sound and it doesn't keep me awake.

It's well known that exposure to too much loud sound may cause damage to hearing, but it's less generally well known in the community, how much is too much. I wish more people understood that damage to hearing comes from both single loud events and from cumulative noise dose. Really it's just like the effects of too much sun. A single instant that causes excessive sunburn can lead to permanent damage. Many people who were exposed to noise through loud machinery or rural work didn't use hearing protection because they didn't realise the damage they were exposing themselves to. However today we understand the damage that loud sound can cause to our hearing, and most people working in background noise use hearing protection. Children at school often don't use hearing protection even though they may be exposed to too much loud sound through a daily combination of activities such as craft and musical instrument practice, coupled with recreational headphone use.

When people who have been gradually losing their hearing or have lost their hearing some time ago first get hearing aids, they sometimes don't understand the world of sounds that they can now experience. Sometimes they're not sure what is noise, and what are soft sounds of speech or other sounds that they have forgotten. When I started wearing my own hearing aids I was surprised at how crunchy the autumn leaves sounded under my feet. At first I thought it must be a particularly crisp autumn. Then I realised I hadn't heard that sound so crisply for a long time and I have only a very mild high-frequency hearing loss. When my husband John started wearing his hearing aids he was surprised to hear some of the engine noises from the car, saying that he had thought that cars just got a lot quieter. We both entered a more colourful hearing world.

I am consistently told how deaf the younger generation are going to be because of the use of headphones. I suspect they will be quite comfortable with using hearing aids when they need them which is more that can be said for 50 to 60 year olds today. For most people, as we get older our hearing deteriorates. Unfortunately it isn't just the mechanism in the ear that deteriorates and it isn't just that sounds get softer. As we get older our auditory memory can deteriorate. When we listen to running speech we hold enough of it in memory at any one time to make sense of whole sentences and blocks of sentences. If I read three sentences from this book aloud to you I'd be hoping that you could store all of that information to understand what I have said. This becomes particularly important when you are listening in noisy or difficult situations. Although we get worse at this we can practice using our auditory memory and researchers believe that this helps us hear better in background noise or other difficult occasions. I do a lot of talk on communication and listening and I usually give people some tips on exercises that they can do or games that they can play to practice improving their auditory memory. There is a commonly used test of auditory memory that you can try with a friend. Ask your partner to recite three non-sequential numbers such as 6, 4 and 9. Your task then is to recite them back but in the reverse order. Keep increasing the length of the number string and see how long the string of numbers is that you can get to.

When we are listening in complex or difficult situations we need to use all our skills and all our engines. And of course we have to use a lot of attention. This can get quite tiring. Sometimes it can seem like too much bother; we lose attention and appear not to hear. The speaker being too far away or having their back to us can create a difficult listening situation. Background interference might just be the kettle boiling. Either way, not hearing in this situation can be interpreted as selective deafness. I spend a lot of time in our hearing clinic helping people overcome the poor communication skills they have developed over the years.

CHAPTER SEVEN

My dad; running, boating and hearing

Sport, science, hearing, and getting involved in trying to make change for the better have long been linked for me. All through my time at the Royal School for the Deaf I was also a track athlete. I belonged to the Derby Ladies Athletics Club.

In the late 1960s, it was less common to be involved in serious sport and training hard, but I had a wonderful coach who was a huge influence in my life. He gave up hours of his personal time to coach kids like me, and it was all voluntary. Richard Dunphy was the most important person in my life, outside of my family. I trained six days a week, often with my dad. Dad went on to become a serious track and field judge. He used to joke that he'd get to the Olympics first, as a judge. Again, he didn't let his hearing stop his participation. Both my parents did a lot to encourage me in athletics. I grew up in an environment where I needed to do my best, whatever that was in, and to pull out energy reserves when the going got tough.

Perhaps my dad's hearing loss gave him extra patience in standing in the quiet by the racetrack on long evenings, as I ran repetition after repetition to get stronger and faster. Alternately, I think he supported me because there was no logical reason why he would not do so. My father was a high achiever in everything he sought to do in his life, even with his hearing deteriorating significantly. He didn't acknowledge his hearing getting in the way. He was an ambitious man and he wanted me to have a good career. In 1960s England, when girls were supposed to have a brief, vocational career, before marriage, my father was on the athletics track with me with a stopwatch and a whistle helping me train and encouraging me to prepare to study science at University. I don't think my father ever came to terms with the woolly nature of girls' education at the time. Girls schooling in England was changing. At school I showed promise in mathematics and sport, and in both pursuits Dad was always there, and I felt I made most progress in both, outside of school. My mother went back to work when I left school, and showed great competence in a leadership role in the administration of a radiotherapy clinic, until then, she'd done what mothers in the 50s and 60s usually did. She brought up the family, and quietly provided the base from which we launched.

On the athletics track, as in life, my father set high standards for me. He never articulated them as high standards. He just set them and it did not occur to me that there were any other standards. And so, on many cold winter evenings (I suppose it was summer sometimes), my father would time my running, in 60 metre blocks, so that I could run 300 metres accurately to a chosen pace. He stood there whilst I did interval training, repeating timed runs of 600 metres, or some other distance, with tiny rests. He probably turned off his hearing aid if I grumbled too much. Being an athlete teaches you that talent isn't enough. Talent gets you started and then it is hours of hard work. I immersed myself in action, to train my body to move fast, and to move well. I also learned the importance of using my brain in sport. Running 400 meters is about running fast, but controlled and tactical. My strategy was to run at a certain pace, and I knew exactly how fast I was running, and then to run the last 100 metres or so, as if I hadn't run anything else. I use that strategy at work today. If I'm feeling tired, I just try to look a little deeper, and pull out some more.

My worlds overlapped. My training partner was Stephen, who was about my age, was deaf, though he had a little hearing. Like many people with severe hearing loss, he used his vision. I was jealous of how well he used his eyes. At the start line, he would pick up cues other than the sound of the gun. He was so visual, he moved on the flash from the gun, while I waited for the bang. I thought he had a bit of an unfair advantage. So, like my dad, Stephen did everything to minimise the chance that his lack of hearing would limit him.

I think Stephen and I were paired up as training partners because we were both a bit different. I was faster than the other girls on the track and my coach thought that pairing me with a boy would push my boundaries physically. It helped Stephen too, because my dad was prepared to put the time in with us both, stop watch and whistle in hand. I guess that Stephen and my dad had a bit of a bond.

In hindsight I suspect that Stephen struggled to fit in. Some of my hearing training mates were not sure about how to interact with him. Occasionally I went to social gatherings with Stephen's friends from his oral school for children who had, what was called, partial hearing. On the way home from these social gatherings, after some time chatting away in the car, I realised that I couldn't talk to Stephen in the car because it was dark, and he couldn't see. In retrospect, I think we both had a soft spot for each other, but neither of us expressed that, and it was partly because casual modes of communication were so different for us both. One of us being deaf and one not, was still too big a difference. I went to see some deaf friends of Stephen's once. His friend, Peter, was partially hearing and used oral language. His wife, Jane was deaf and signed. Peter wouldn't allow his wife to sign to their hearing child, in case their child failed to learn good speech. Jane's isolation from her child, and her child from Jane was heartbreaking to witness. This was the result of the polarising education system that prevailed well into the 1970s.

I contacted Stephen and asked him to update me on the last 30 years of his life. He said:

'I am vice chairman of Bridport Deaf Club. I also have a cochlear implant in my left ear, for which this was done at Southampton, while I was there I had been asking for you, and no-one knew of you… Also for some unknown reason, last February/March 2013 I lost my hearing in my right ear, after having four coughs, colds and sore throats, in quick succession, I put my hearing aid on that morning and could not hear, my wife Alison asked what was I was doing, I explained that my hearing aid was not working, she said "yes it is I can hear it whistling!"'

Sadly, his hearing had got much worse, perhaps because of a viral infection, associated with the cold. It seems recurrent virus's of some kind had taken the rest of his vulnerable hearing.

My father managed extraordinarily well with his hearing loss, but his hobbies were typically rather solitary. Like me he was very fond of sailing. I was cruising around the Wooden Boat forums one evening, recently, rather nostalgically, and couldn't believe my eyes when I saw a reference to my hearing aid company (Blamey Saunders). This was so wonderful, because, I went into hearing and hearing aid research, inspired by my dad, whose passion was wooden boats. I was too involved with study, work and track athletics to get involved in boating, but I absorbed a love of the water from dad.

Many holidays involved hiring some kind of boat, and spending time admiring and coveting beautiful boats. While I was studying at University I was also a member of the British Ocean Youth Club – a wonderful experience that took me sailing on large ketches, and emphasised team work and hard work. What a wonderful organisation. Later, I crewed on a racing National 18, mostly in the Solent, for Ross Coles, a professor of hearing research and the son of the fabled ocean racer and prolific author, Adlard Coles. In my dad's life, there were always boats, and there was always woodwork, so they were bound to come together. He built some fine, award winning model boats.

DAD'S LESSONS ON HEARING AND LISTENING WITH A HEARING LOSS

Dad took early retirement, probably in part because of his hearing loss, to run a boat chartering business on the river Dart. He was known locally as 'Saunders of the River'. Customers wanted to rent comfortable, motorised gin palaces, rather than character filled, enthusiasts boats, so he rented out motorised gin palaces, but for his own pleasure, he sailed a Drascombe Lugger, and in his spare time made wooden boats. By the time Dad was in his late 40s he was very deaf, and totally dependent on his hearing aid, which frankly in the 1970s was not very good. But boating was kind to him. The water, the fresh air, the peace and the interaction with the boat – his hearing aid was probably turned off half the time.

Now I know more about hearing and listening, I think of all those beautiful coastal river sounds that he probably never heard, like the haunting sound of the curlew, the lap of water against the boat… Meanwhile, I had graduated from quantum physics and studied audiology and hearing science, and began an adventurous career, which was supposed to include sailing round the world, but so far hasn't. But I'm happy to have helped many people hear well. I've worked in cochlear implant research and development. Sadly my adored father died before I got into research in that area, and it's disappointing that he couldn't benefit from the work I did. I've moved on from cochlear implants, to hearing aids, and hearing aids have got better partly because of cochlear implant research. I've played a small part in that – small in that there are many, many researchers; large in that, my business partner Peter and I have taken the technology to create better and more accessible hearing aids. Inspired by my dad's example to self-manage his hearing aids, we have designed hearing aids that are so smart and so simple to set up that people can easily do it themselves. To make it easier still, we've designed a very informative and helpful hearing test that can be done at home, too. It doesn't need a soundproof room and lots of expensive equipment. My dad, the engineer, would have had a great time, setting up his hearing aids, so that sounds were as he wanted. He wouldn't even have had to leave his boat. No long trips to the hearing aid centre, no waiting. Not everyone is as independent as my dad was, so we've made sure that we also provided a remote audiology service, accessible on the Internet. Untreated hearing loss leads to other problems, including accelerating cognitive decline. My dad tried hard with his hearing aids, but he never had access to the type of hearing aid technology we have today. Hearing aids have changed enormously in the last 20 years.

My dad died in 1997, after a longish illness. Before he died he started to write a book about his hearing. He's the first of my hero stories in this book. Dad seemed to hear extraordinarily well for the small amount of hearing he actually had, and his book left me with insights into how he really managed to communicate. He relied a lot on reading lips, watching faces and using context. Everyone, even with good hearing uses those cues, but people without much hearing generally use them more. Humans are programmed to use listen with hearing, vision and attention. My father was using good, and very well practiced listening skills to communicate.

In his book about his experiences, he wrote,

'Many films achieve effects by presenting speech with the speaker off-screen, or with the head turned away, presumably for artistic reasons. It is arguable that the art is not well served if the accompanying dialogue is unintelligible to a sizable section of the

audience, but you may expect some difficulty in comprehension when this happens and it is not unlike watching a film in a foreign language.'

In my hearing aid clinic today, and through my communication with people online or by phone, I hear or read this observation all the time, even if they have relatively good hearing aids. There are other gadgets that help make the speech clearer, but, even with good hearing aids, or some kind of special TV gadget, it's a good idea to use all the cues you can to make life easier, and so that you don't have to concentrate so hard. The chances are that your fellow viewers will be glad you switched them on, because they're probably having trouble too. Just try not to laugh or be too distracted, when the subtitle says 'spooky flute music'.

My father had advice for other people too: He wrote, 'It does not pay to keep your hearing aid a secret – rather the reverse in fact.'

This is a great thing to say. If you're reading this and thinking 'that's crazy', think again. I'm always surprised that there is a market for deep-in-the ear canal, invisible hearing aids. There's no evidence to say they are better than good quality little hearing aids that sit just behind the ear, but the wearer has turned off the visible signs that might have caused other people to be helpful. Especially for older people, hearing aids don't do the whole job of correcting speech recognition when the conditions for hearing are difficult, so it's helpful to have other people cooperate by looking at you and speaking nice and clearly, without you having to tell them. Most people would welcome being given a seat on the tram if you are in need. Take the helping hand, and don't hide the hearing loss.

My father wrote later, 'The job of interpreting conversation is that much more difficult if the talkers head is turned away. It is surprising how much reliance is put on a small element of lip reading even by normal hearing people.'

And of course, he's right. We have four engines for speech recognition;

two ears and two eyes, and we have an amazing central processing unit, called the brain, that puts the information together. Everyone notices when the audio and the visual aren't synchronised properly in a film. That's a clear example of being wired to use both senses. Sound gets softer as you move further from the source. The measured sound level obeys the inverse square law. The inverse square law predicts the first estimate of the sound you would get at a point that's away from the sound source, if you are in a reasonably open area. However, if you are in an area with reflective surfaces, the law breaks down.

We might think of two different sorts of noise – one you may be able to control, and one you can't. The decibel level is reduced by about 6 dB, every time you double the distance between the listener and the sound source. This is because intensity is reduced to a quarter of the original.

Imagine you are going shopping and you and your friend are in the kitchen. Your friend is reciting the shopping list to you as you walk away. You move away by half a meter and the voice level is half as loud. That's a lot! The listener is probably not facing the speaker any more either. Consider that many consonants are less than half as loud as vowels. If the later items in the list contain consonants, you may be doomed to be reprimanded for not listening properly and making mistakes. The sound picture of cheese and peas are near enough that chopping the loudness in half and taking away the visual cue could lead you to a platter of peas and biscuits at dinner.

Excellent hearing aids should keep sound audible and comfortable, which helps, but, my advice is to stay standing still and listen to the whole list before you move away – even with your hearing aids on. It will help to watch the speaker too.

CHAPTER EIGHT

ICE-CREAMS AND
HEARING TESTS

My search for answers didn't take me to an Indian Ashram or to Rome, although I did think about the Greek Islands once. A year in hearing services in London, rather then a year in Provence, made me realise that I didn't want to be a Senior Expert on such a weak base of knowledge and experience. I'd done a pretty good job so far, but I didn't feel that I was the whole package that such a role really deserved. I thought I'd end up facing a lack of basic knowledge somewhere in the years ahead. So, I decided to leave the swish surrounds of the new Charing Cross Hospital, with its swimming pool, its squash courts and its parties in the mortuary. I had completed a Master's degree in Audiology as preparation to take up a role as an Audiological Scientist, in the British NHS. I did a reasonable job at Charing Cross Hospital, I believe, but I was hungry to study further and I was offered a Research Fellowship at Southampton University in the Institute for Sound and Vibration Research (ISVR0), still one of the most prestigious places in the world to study hearing. The head of the unit was well-known professor of audiology Ross Coles. Ross Coles was a leading researcher in audiology in the late 1970s, he had been successful in obtaining grant funding for a research project that would investigate why some deaf children learned to speak better than others. This was to be my project. We were still in the pre-cochlear implant era. In audiology though, technology had recently taken a jump forward, with the development of auditory electro-physiology testing. I was about to become an early researcher and expert in this topic. At this time children diagnosed with hearing loss were usually classified as being hearing impaired without regard to the potential site of the auditory dysfunction, and the hearing loss was characterised only by its extent. Depending on the age of diagnosis some measure of speech processing and ability to discriminate speech sounds may have been made. It turns out that Ross was right, although I didn't demonstrate it in my PhD. More sensitive equipment available today, has led to the identification of a condition called auditory neuropathy, where a child isn't able to process the incoming sound properly. The sound coded in the cochlear, doesn't get transmitted up the auditory pathway properly.

Speech recognition and understanding is a complex process. Otherwise it would have been easier to develop artificial speech recognition. Human beings have the ability to understand speech and language in quite difficult conditions. We have the ability to pick one conversation at a background of other speech; we have the ability to understand speakers even though their pronunciation is sloppy or their accent is unfamiliar to us; we have the ability to determine meaning from complex patterns of sound. We can do all this because we have the ability in the auditory periphery to detect and code complex patterns and then our hearing nerve pathways convey the information hearing centres in the brain. There is interaction with attention, and with visual pathways and visual processing. Even young children routinely use lip-reading to help them. Here English speakers have a well-tuned auditory visual path to understanding speech. Adults first notice hearing deterioration when the going is tough. We first have problems when the listening conditions are difficult. This can be due to the peripheral detection system becoming less functional, or to some decline in the central process, or both. At the time of my PhD I thought it was important to find out which. With children, it probably is; however with adults it matters less, as the remediation is probably the same either way.

When I took this work on in the late 70s, audiology was still fairly new in its applications with deaf children, in England. It was much more established in the US. At that time, children were categorised for education placement, largely, by the extent of their audiogram (degree of hearing loss as measured by the beep test), but researchers and educators were worried as to why some children didn't learn oral language, despite hearing aids and audiometric assessment. Researchers were worried about the findings of the Warnock report (1978): this was a report of the committee of enquiry into the education of handicapped children and young people in England. The focus of the report was on the inclusion of children with disabilities into mainstream education, that is, children with a disability should be in ordinary classrooms but with extra support. This report threw up a lot of issues in the area of deaf education, already strongly factionalised between methods of teaching and communicating.

By the time I started this research study, there were some suggestions from other research that children who had additional processing problems more centrally in the auditory system may have additional perceptual deficit which could be sufficient to slow down their linguistic cognitive or other educational progress. It had already been ascertained that this could occur as a result of not being able to process rapidly presented signals that form the basis of speech sounds. It could be due to the nerve fibres not firing in synchrony. Research in the last few years has shown I was on the right track, but without sufficiently sensitive equipment, and that there is indeed a hearing condition called auditory neuropathy. But I didn't discover it, and some scientists were sceptical of my efforts to try. The new auditory electro-physiology techniques held strong possibility to be able to shed light on this area. In the late 1970s, although the central auditory processors had been determined, the neurological basis and the location for central processing of speech were not fully understood. At the time I started my research, scientists were not entirely clear as to which structures in the brain stem and the brain, after the point at which the input from two ears was combined, were most important for speech processing. It was an ideal to have meaningful information about the status of the central auditory and speech processing pathways to implement an effective remediation program. However, we had neither strong knowledge, nor the measurement method. Today, we have a somewhat, though not full, understanding of the central hearing pathways and speech perception mechanism, and we can measure much more, but we are a long way from being able to provide all the information for therapeutic information that is sought.

Even in the late 1970s behavioural tests existed to investigate central auditory dysfunction. However at this time they were considered relatively experimental and we did not have access to comprehensive sets of normal data. Additionally such data as there was had been collected from children who did not have raised hearing thresholds or hearing impairment. The children I wanted to investigate belonged to a subgroup of the population of children who exhibited receptive language disorders and had hearing loss.

So, I started on the next stage of my career and education in hearing and the results of hearing loss as a Research Fellow in a prestigious research institution, and crewing for a well-known and experienced sailor. How lucky was I? There, at the University, I did a lot of research in fundamental techniques in auditory evoked potentials, which was a young science at the time. My interest, however, lay in the potential for using these new techniques to improve the life of children with hearing loss. It was clear that they were going to have a useful role in diagnostic audiology too.

Auditory evoked potential are very small bursts of electrical activity (voltage potentials) that occur as a result of sound stimuli, and that can be measured to reveal a lot about the state of the hearing nerve pathways and the brain. They were discovered in the early part of the 20th century, but the first commercial system for recording them was produced in 1970, and this first machine was discontinued only three years later due to an inappropriate choice of recording parameters. The responses are recording of electrical activity from the skin surface, in response to a sound stimulus. In other words, the ear hears a sound, and electrodes are used to track its passage to the brain. If no sound is heard, there will be no response. When a nerve receives the signal, the response is very small, so there are technical challenges in demonstrating the response, which are overcome with computational averaging methods.

The preparatory work for evoked potentials could be traced back to Galvani's discovery of the electrical activity of biological tissue in 1790. Galvani's discovery that the muscles of dead frog's legs twitched with a spark was only a chance observation, but this is the kind of observation that is so important in the history of science.

Galvani was really investigating something else at the time – his dinner. There were implications for the history of electricity, which his friend and colleague Volta investigated, but Galvani investigated further, and decided that the muscle contractions were actually caused by the flow of electricity in the frog. He theorised that a 'nervo-electric' fluid was conducted from the nerves to the muscle, causing the contraction. Today we're able to record this burst of electrical energy.

A hundred years later the Liverpool physician, Richard Caton, demonstrated to the British Medical Association (1875) that electrical potentials could be recorded from the brains of rabbits and monkeys and that these potentials varied over time. The Electrocortiograms, as these measurements became known, were first photographically recorded by Pravdich Neminsky in 1913, using a string galvanometer. Following this, discoveries came thick and fast, laying the foundations for today's knowledge of auditory evoked potentials.

In 1929, the German psychiatrist, Hans Berger, demonstrated recordings of the first human electroencephalogram (EEG) from scalp electrodes, and the following year he reported a change in the rhythm from a sleeping volunteer, following presentation of a loud noise. He called this measure, the 'K' complex. Berger's work on the EEG was part of a 40-year study in psychophysical research.

The K complex was later renamed by Hallowell Davis (1896-1992), as the 'V' potential. Hallowell Davis and his wife, Nancy, later took me, a humble early-career researcher, out for dinner in St. Louis, and treated me with the civility that one might expect to be reserved for famous scientists. Hallowell Davis was one of the first people in the USA to have his own encephalography (EEG) recorded. He also made a significant contribution to our understanding of hearing by showing that hair cells in the inner ear play an important role in transforming the mechanical stimulus of sound into electrical impulses that can be processed by the brain. Davis didn't just 'rename' the K complex; he identified the important all-or-none characteristics of the auditory nerve impulses in 1926, he also helped us understand the contributions from the cochlear itself and from the hearing nerve. Ernest Wever and Charles Bray impressively demonstrated the waveform replicating properties of the cochlear microphonic potential in 1930. Their work, rather improbably, showed initial results in a technique now known as the Cat Telephone, where they had wired a live cat into a telephone system and replayed the output. The electrical potentials that they recorded demonstrate that bursts of electrical activity transmit sounds to the brain, and the particular potential they recorded is now known was the Wever-Bray effect. Hallowell Davis demonstrated that this potential had two components, the cochlear microphonic and the auditory nerve potential. But there are more, and surprising findings.

We now understand that the cochlear microphonic is a receptor potential believed to be generated primarily by outer hair cells, in the cochlear. Where the potential is intact and other signs of cochlear function are normal (oto-acoustic emissions, that were not known of when I did my research), and neural responses are not, then there is some basis for assigning the interpretation of auditory neuropathy – a condition where a problem in the auditory nerve causes a kind of central auditory hearing loss. Oto-acoustic emissions are interesting in their own right.

When I was in Southampton, working on my PhD, I met a researcher called David Kemp, who was working at London University and associated with the Royal National Throat, Nose and Ear Hospital at Gray's Inn Road, (founded in 1874). He demonstrated the oto-acoustic emission, which became known as 'The Kemp Echo'. To be there at one of his early demonstrations was amazing.

Oto-acoustic emissions are sounds spontaneously generated from the hair cells in the ear. In response to a sound stimulus, it appears that outer hair cells in the cochlea have an amplifying effect (now known as the 'cochlear amplifier') and if a very short sound is presented to the ear, so that the response is synchronised, then the resulting motion in the cochlea, actually creates sounds that can be recorded by a microphone fitted into the ear canal. The eardrum gets vibrations that have been transmitted backwards through the middle ear. Dr Kemp set up a system to demonstrate the effect and put an amplifier and loudspeaker in the set up, so that we could easily hear the ear hearing. It was definitely one of those 'wow, you needed to be there' moments. Because the ear activity could be measured, it had the potential to become used as a measure of cochlear health. The cochlear amplifier contributes to our hearing sensitivity. The OEA's as they have become abbreviated to, have become part of objective hearing testing.

The individual's ear responses are so unique, they are like a fingerprint, and some researchers think they could be used for personal security. Perhaps you will one day put on headphones, and hear a sound, and the 'hearing print' will be used to let you into your computer. Tricky if you have a cold with blocked ears, as this would likely effect the hearing response or 'ear-print'.

There was an American composer called Maryanne Amacher who worked extensively with oto-acoustic emissions. She composed several 'ear dances' designed to stimulate 'third tones' coming from the ears themselves. Her music is extraordinary. She did a number of site-specific pieces, but there are recordings of her work that give some insight into how she played with physiology and acoustics to create very unusual effects. You need good quality speakers and it doesn't work with headphones. Anyway, suffice it to say that when I first heard the Kemp Echo in a lecture demonstration, I was almost disbelieving – yet now it is routinely used as a way to monitor hearing function.

It seems that there are two types of hair cells in the ear commonly called the inner and outer hair cells. Outer hair cells help the inner hair cells sense soft sounds. Outer hair cells are the ones that get damaged, in general, by wear and tear, so when the inner hair cells are damaged as well, this is likely to be caused by events beyond wear and tear, such as ageing or the effects of noise, illness or drugs. Hearing loss is greater than if it was outer hair cell damage alone. If hearing loss is up to about 50 dB loss at a particular frequency, then the cause is probably due to damage to the outer air cell: if it's greater than 50 dB then the loss is probably due to both inner and outer hair cells. When I look at hearing test results and see the big change from less than 50 dB hearing loss to more than 50 dB hearing loss over a small frequency range then I wonder what is going on in the cochlea, because we don't know. In

1926 Hallowell Davis identified the important all-or-none characteristics of the auditory nerve impulses, and demonstrated that the hearing potential had two components, the cochlear microphonic and the auditory nerve potential. This was the first demonstration that you could identify responses from the nerve and from the cochlea separately, and has become quite important in the diagnosis of different types of hearing disorder.

We now understand that the cochlear microphonic is a receptor potential believed to be generated primarily by outer hair cells, in the cochlear. Where the potential is intact, and neural responses are not, then there is some basis for a diagnosis of auditory neuropathy – a condition where a problem in the auditory nerve causes some kind of central auditory hearing loss. This has been a step forward in understanding why some children don't do well with hearing aids.

I discussed my thesis with Hallowell Davis, and he said he thought it most unlikely that I would find any central auditory abnormalities, using evoked potentials. Professor Davis said that he thought that my hypothesis was flawed, and that other neurological signs would accompany any such central auditory problems. He was both right and wrong, in that we both underestimated the technical feasibility of recording the cochlear microphonic, and hence it's potential importance in understanding hearing disorders. In science and technology we have to be careful not to let current knowledge constrain our thinking.

When I look back on my PhD work today, I can see it as a snapshot in time. Auditory evoked potentials were a new tool. Opinions on deaf education were polarised. Cochlear implants were still in development. Within a few years, the pace of development in computing changed the landscape forever, to the extent that I didn't bother to publish from my PhD.

Hearing loss has typically been measured by putting a pair of headphones on to someone, sitting them in a quiet room and then finding out what the soft sound is that they can hear. It can be quite a difficult task to do with children. Depending on their age or temperament they may be unable or unwilling to participate. The result of the hearing test is a map of the softest sounds that someone can hear at particular frequencies. The frequencies tested are typically from 250 Hz, which is near middle C, up in octave intervals to 8000 Hz. Those frequencies are considered to be the ones most important for hearing speech. The degree of hearing loss measured in this way gives only a very broad indication for future successes in acquiring oral language in the absence of say a cochlear implant. The tester, or educator, used to make assumptions concerning which features of the speech spectrum would be perceived based on the audiometric configuration. This doesn't tell you much about the effect that degree of hearing loss has on other aspects of perception, such as the ability to discriminate between sounds of different frequencies, temporal timing, coding ability, ability to code intensity, and the processes occurring to code and interpret sound centrally. In the late 1970s, researchers had not shown a good relationship between even direct measures of hearing for speech sounds, with spoken language ability. There were some good experimental studies investigating the effect of degrees of hearing loss on language development. Differences in the experimental results were due, in part, to the different experimental methods that were used, and to the selection of very different groups of study participants. The dilemmas in measurement methods pushed researchers to making over simplified categories for children on hearing and speech abilities.

In the late 70s, I had a hypothesis that it might be possible to predict which children would learn oral language and which wouldn't on the basis of a set of tests with electrodes on their scalp listening to the clicks and tones. You don't have to be a hearing scientist or educator to work out that the child's language and understanding was probably influenced by their environment, their upbringing, and the type of language they had been taught especially in an era when some children used spoken language whether they could hear or not and some children signed. My challenge was to find a group of children who had rather similar if not identical environments. Here I was helped by the head teacher of Woodford School in Essex, England. It was a boarding school where children were required to be aural/oral; that is to talk and they were not allowed to sign. I have read accounts on the Internet from some of the children, that the educational regime was not pleasant. However, the school opened their arms to me and I spent many weeks at the school testing all kinds of skills with the children from their ability to read to other psychological and educational measures. The children ranged in age from six to 16, and they'd leave their class to come and do my puzzles and tests. But to do my sophisticated testing of auditory evoked potentials at that time, I needed a bigger and specialised test set up. Today this equipment is available with a laptop computer. But then, the children came to me at Southampton General Hospital in the University wing to do these mysterious tests.

At that time the hospital had one of the best canteens and catering facilities I have ever come across in a hospital. They had a formal dining room; a healthy salad bar; a traditional type of canteen but best of all they had a hamburger bar. For me this was a treat that I could give the children. This was the highlight of the day for them. When the testing was finished we all bundled into my car and we would go down to the pier at Southampton. We'd all walk along to the end and have the most enormous ice creams that we could find before the children went back on the train. Some of the children in my study, were as young as six. For the research, I needed to stick several small circular disc electrodes on to the child's scalp. Then they were required to lie quiet and relaxed for about an hour and a half while my testing went on. The testing involved hearing interminable chains of clicking noises. It can be fairly challenging to make six-year-old boys lie still and relaxed for around an hour and half listening to nothing more interesting than sounds repeating like the sounds of a thousand cicadas. On the whole the children were astonishing. I can only think that the carers must have really prepared them well. One boy went back to school and made up a lot of stories about pain and blood which made it a little bit challenging for the little girl who came down the next day. But apart from that slight glitch we got through a lot of data collection and had quite a lot of fun.

In contrast, I don't think the school was a very happy place. Can you imagine not being able to hear or speak clearly, in a way that other people can understand? I needed to quantify how well the children could communicate, and since these children, for better or worse, were being trained to communicate orally (talking), I thought the best way to assess this ability was directly, so I decided to record both oral reading and conversational samples of speech from the children. The most common strategy to evaluate speech intelligibility is to use panels of judges to rate the intelligibility of the speech. I recorded 20-second samples of speech from each child. They read from a short, familiar page, drawn from classroom material, and after discussion with their teacher. Most of the recordings were hard to understand.

While I was busy trying to find out why some deaf children didn't manage to learn clear spoken language, and others did, I was also trying to find out how much being able to hear high pitches outside the area, more typically known as the speech frequencies, helped children with otherwise poor hearing. I had two groups of children under test. My second group of children were local, and were children in schools that provided facilities for those with some useable hearing – what we used to call 'Partial Hearing Units'. I asked teachers to identify children, who they thought were doing particularly well considering their measured hearing loss. I took these children and tested their hearing with the equipment I had to test hearing outside of the normal range. This was where the work that I did on testing children without hearing problems came in as the baseline. That was only ever going to tell me part of the story.

The audiogram has a worldwide history originating in the field of otology during the late 19th century and migrating to the profession of audiology after the Second World War. It typically offers a visual base by which hearing sensitivity is presented, judged, and compared to previous other recordings. As a tool documenting hearing sensitivity, only the audiogram grid component must adhere to one of two formal standards that are dictated by ANSI or ASHA.

Dr Charles Berlin was a leading professor of audiology at the Kresge Institute in New Orleans. In 1978 he published a most interesting study that showed that children who had hearing in the frequencies above 4 kHz, which is better than their hearing at lower frequencies, then use it, and it seems to help the intelligibility of their speech. So, I decided to test the hearing of the children in my study at 12 kHz and at 16 kHz. It seemed possible that if there were any children in my group who had particularly clear speech, that this could be an explanation. There was only one problem. When I was doing my PhD work there was not standardised equipment available to do the tests. Part of the reason for the shortage of equipment was the difficulty in calibrating. I needed something to produce sounds of a high enough frequency and I needed headphones that were good enough to produce the high frequency tones. There weren't any commercial systems that were set up to measure high frequencies, so I set up an audiometer myself that would work at higher frequencies. I didn't have any research funds to go out and buy lots of headphones, so I set up the best calibration and measurement system that I could, and decided to find a way to source and calibrated the right headphones. I went to a top Hi-Fi shop and convinced them to lend me one of every pair of their top headphones; I can't remember how many shops I went to before someone agreed to that proposition. I thought it was a pretty good deal for the shop – look at all that useful scientific data I could supply. They didn't seem very convinced. Anyway, I evaluated all the headphones, and found the money from somewhere to buy the best pair. I gave the shop the test results, and everyone was happy in the end.

I also needed normal hearing people to standardise the system. Where was I going to get people with normal hearing at 16 kHz, when we have done all our best hearing before we are aged ten? The answer was clear. I needed children. The children needed to be otologically normal. Samuel Rosen and his colleagues studied children in Sudan from two different backgrounds. One group were from the Mabaan tribe and another group were from city children. They showed that noise seemed to have damaged the hearing in the youngest group (10–18). This is something for us to consider today, as children are exposed to so much noise.

Finding 20 otologically normal children to take part in an experiment, when you are a University researcher, in an engineering faculty, isn't all that easy. Happily for me, the parents of the children said I could test their children. Better than that, they let me collect them from the holiday play scheme, and take them in the back of my little white mini van (I did have carpet on the floor) back to the University to test. I'd zoom to the next suburb, collect two children;, zoom back to the University, check their ears, and if they were suitable, test their hearing at the high test frequencies, and standard frequencies as well, and then zoom back with them – via the ice-cream shop, according to my unusual PhD protocol. In this way, I established normal values for our ability to hear high frequencies.

CHAPTER NINE

I'VE COME TO LOOK FOR AMERICA

By this time, I had studied enough to believe that we in Britain were falling behind in the use of contemporary techniques to assess children's hearing. I was one of the people in Britain who was leading in the knowledge of assessment of children's hearing. I wanted to learn first hand from the experience and research that I had read about in the United States. Audiology was a more mature profession at that point in the United States. I applied for a Churchill Fellowship, from the Winston Churchill Memorial Trust, to visit America to study the assessment of children's hearing. I put together a dream study tour with a who's who of audiology heroes and then applied for the fellowship. The application was like a grant proposal. My initial goal was to get an interview, and I did. When I went to interview, I had arrived at a sombre looking office in Whitehall, London. The room was big, and mostly full of table. There were several people on the interview panel, all in suits. I have to say I felt nervous, and I wasn't sure in which direction to look. The interviewers were spread all around this giant table. A friendly voice said: 'Tell us about what you want to do.' To my surprise the voice belonged to Joyce Grenfell. Although Joyce Grenfell had many talents and a diverse career I was most familiar with the monologues about young children that she recorded. My mother had a number of her humorous recordings. Joyce was a wonderful interviewer, and put me at sufficient ease to talk with enthusiasm about my ambitions.

Major-General Lascelles was director-general of the Winston Churchill Memorial Trust, at the time I applied. I was home in Derby, when my mother excitedly called that the Queen's cousin was on the phone and wanted to talk to me. This seemed highly unlikely, as I was not aware they had any connections with royalty. However the result of my phone call was that I had been awarded the fellowship, I was off to America to learn more about hearing and testing children's hearing. The fellowship was extremely well managed, and the grant advisors were keen to ensure that I had sufficient funds and would be able to complete my goals.

I started my fellowship in Pennsylvania at Temple University. This was my first trip to the USA and the scientists and clinicians that I went to see were keen to make sure I had a good cultural start as well as a good professional start. Temple University was already famous for its food trucks, but this was a new experience to me. I returned to the laboratory complete with a large assortment of delicious, unhealthy comfort food, consolidating my view that I had come to the land of chips and hamburgers. One of my academic hosts had welcomed me into their home, which was a large and beautiful home in Westchester. This was picture book America – large homes dotted across the rolling hills, with no boundary fences. Back at Temple, I saw a less affluent side of life. Until then, my experience of health care was the British National Health Service where everyone had access to care. Whilst at Temple University, I saw the use of automated electro-physiology testing; this is what I had come to see. It's a good technique to use when it's hard to get cooperation from the child. The child being tested was an intellectually disabled African American girl. The goal was to find out how well, or how poorly, she could hear. Electro-physiology tests are quite time consuming. The child clearly had a hearing loss and I expected that we would find out how bad it was. However, the audiologist stopped before they had detailed information. They could have spent longer, and got a more precise result, but I was told that there were no funds for her to have hearing aids, or therapy, so it wasn't necessary. I was stunned. This wouldn't happen in Britain, under the NHS. It was the first time I truly appreciated how wonderful it was to have universal health care. Earlier in the day, I had been driven through areas of North Philadelphia that also shocked me. I went through an area that was almost entirely African Americans. It was very run down, and showed signs of high unemployment, from the number of people sitting around: like many things on my trip, it left a big impression.

In total contrast, I visited the Children's Hospital of Philadelphia. It's a hospital with a long history of medical leadership and excellence. With the exception of Charing Cross Hospital in London I was most accustomed to old Victorian hospitals. The Children's Hospital of Philadelphia was magnificent. We drove into the hospital department in the basement carpark. We went up in the lift and entered the hospital foyer which was very brightly painted, and walked through a beautiful courtyard. There were trees in this light and airy courtyard, and there was seating laid out as though it was a pleasant park. I think what chiefly impressed me about the Children's Hospital of Philadelphia was that it was so light and airy after the old Victorian hospitals that I was used to in Britain. All the corridors were modern, clean, smart, comfortable and most of all cheerful.

I had of course come to learn more about the testing of hearing. This was my first experience of working with a very diverse multidisciplinary team. It was a clear demonstration of the importance of professionals with different expertise working well together. I have encountered many bad examples of this since, which is very sad. The experience at the Children's Hospital in Philadelphia left me with an ideal that the child should be absolutely at the centre of their assessments and the professionals should coordinate each other to be able to give the best advice and treatment. Because hearing and listening in communication involves the ear and the brain it is particularly important that psychologists, educationalists, speech therapists and audiologists work well together. I fear that sometimes, even today, specialists don't see outside of their narrow discipline and that works to the disadvantage of the child or indeed any patient in a medical system.

One of the things that I particularly liked about the assessment of hearing in this environment, at the Children's Hospital, was the audiologists use of informal observations. The audiologist had music playing as the child entered the assessment suite, and he carefully watched the child's behaviour as he walked in, and heard the music. This observation gave the audiologist insight that the child could react to the sound. He had quite a lot of hearing. It sounds very simple. It may be done in many places today but I had never seen that technique used before. My studies at the University of Southampton were leading to a growing interest in the processes that occur in the nervous system, between the ear and the brain, and indeed to what occurs in the brain itself, in response to sound. The techniques I saw at the Children's Hospital integrated studies around hearing and listening and language and provided me with some strong perspectives to take forward. In this environment any children with language and learning disorders were assessed using a neuro metric test battery. They had quite sophisticated equipment. I'm amused that in my notes of that visit, I said that I was becoming converted to the concept of total communication deaf children. Total communication is the term given to children who use both oral communication and sign. It's substantially accepted today as a normal way if teaching and learning. Clearly it was so controversial when I was in America that I documented my own changing thoughts.

The rest of the time at Temple was spent with leading researchers, clinicians, lecturers and PhD students. I also saw a very high level of rigour and competency in the approach to clinical training, which was to serve me well when I was arranging clinical placements, or hosting student clinicians later in my career. I also became acquainted with the political professional issues, which led to the formation of the American Academy of Audiology not many years later.

From Philadelphia I went to Ottawa to learn more about techniques of auditory electro-physiology. This time I was visiting a laboratory not the clinic, but the scientists were interested in finding out more about what they called perceptual disorders rather than auditory disorders. Auditory electro-physiology was still a fairly young science and clinical technique. I was interested in some of the 'nerdier' aspects to do with the actual recording techniques. My next stop was Chicago. I had particularly wanted to visit Northwestern University, which we might regard as the birthplace of audiology education. More than the science and the audiology I think I was impressed with the magnificent location on the shores of Lake Michigan. I spent some time at Northwestern meeting with a variety of researchers from different academic areas. It was an enlightening opportunity, to think about the whole communication process in an environment where I could ask leading researchers questions. I spent a lot of time here, pondering about measurement procedure and how the techniques used for a particular test, actually influence the results you measure. The quantum physicist in me should not have been surprised. I also watched some clinical evaluations and learned a little about the challenge of getting the balance right between supervising students and being a good clinician.

I don't remember exactly where I was staying in Chicago except that it was near rapid transit system the 'L', and that was how I got about town. I think that prior to going to Chicago all I knew of the city itself was gleaned from gangster movies so I was prepared to be uncomfortable there. It turned out that Men in Black carrying violin cases did not patrol the streets. However the note on the back of my hotel door advised that I should not leave the hotel alone, and an unfortunate encounter with a taxi driver did not increase my confidence or sense of safety. This was 1979, the city was drab and I felt it was decaying a little. It was 12 years before I would be back and the change was indescribable. I thoroughly enjoyed my second visit to Chicago, years later.

Somewhere in the trip I took a bus to Buffalo where I went out for brunch with students from the audiology course at the University of Buffalo. I had just called their Department office, and was met with a kind invitation to meet the students. This was a pattern that has been repeated on my professional travels, over the years. I have received much kind and generous hospitality. My main reason for wanting to visit Buffalo was to use the weekend to go to Niagara Falls. I have never been very good at taking time off whilst working overseas, but I was certainly glad that I spent the weekend in Buffalo and at the Niagara Falls.

My next stop was to Professor Hallowell Davis in St Louis. He was effectively the inventor of the EEG. This was like meeting audiology royalty. Davis took my PhD research studies very seriously and gave me considered replies to all my questions. I hope that through my career I have given as much serious attention to young people near the beginning of their career, as he did.

St Louis was and still is home to the Central Institute for the Deaf. CID, as it is commonly known, is primarily an oral school for deaf children. Hallowell Davis was Director of the associated research Institute. It's had more recent publicity when school graduate, Heather Whitestone-McCallum became the first deaf woman to be crowned Miss America in 1995.

The next highlight came with my visit to the Centre for Communication Disorders at Boys Town, Nebraska. Father Edward Flanagan purchased

Overlook farm, on the edge of Omaha, Nebraska, and moved the boys from the orphanage that he had founded a few years earlier to live there. The farm subsequently became known as the 'Village of Boys Town'. It later became enormously famous after a movie was made about it, where Spencer Tracey played Father Flanagan. The publicity helped raise sufficient funds to launch the Boy's Town National Research Hospital, which specialised in services for children with hearing and speech disorders. When I visited, children would come from a wide geographical area. The goal was to establish a diagnosis for their communication disorder and to provide a treatment plan that they could take away with them. The structure at that time was divided into research, medical, audiological and learning disabilities. It was early recognition of the relationship between learning disabilities and more subtle communication disorders. This is an area that is problematic for parents and educators today.

Once again, the beauty of the environment struck me. This was another stark contrast to the old institutions that I had been accustomed to in Britain. I remember entering the building and seeing a large round colourful couch. The attending child went into a waiting playroom. No time was wasted, while the child was waiting and playing he or she was observed through a one-way glass window. The waiting playroom was small but thoughtfully constructed of slopes little stairways and tiny doors. The medical work was done first. I recall state of the art Ear, Nose and Throat facilities with any necessary head and neck x-rays carried out nearby. The audiology assessment suites were hidden behind brightly painted doors. The area for 'automatic auditory evoked potential testing' was separate and very comfortable. The programme for the child was coordinated by an educationalist; a teacher of the deaf in fact. This was my first encounter with the divide in the approach to children with communication disorders or learning difficulties.

My experience to date shows that all around the world cases may be steered, either, through a medically oriented program or through an educationally oriented program. I have seen many examples in Australia of children who appear to be having specific difficulties perhaps hearing in background noise; perhaps other classroom difficulties and not being evaluated by this team approach. The results vary, but sadly include; misdiagnosis, inappropriate and narrow labelling; lack of a constructive and therapeutic path forward and parental confusion. As an audiologist, I am familiar with the area of central auditory processing disorder. I was trying to evaluate that in my research studies using auditory evoked potentials, but I couldn't get past the fact that the children in my studies were dominated by large hearing losses. This isn't always the case, but the story of ear meets brain is influenced by other factors such as attention, and I believe that parents of children with that diagnosis make sure that all factors have been considered, and that there are therapeutic strategies to help.

I am so glad I had that experience at Boys Town, to see what can be done when a comprehensive team works together. Because the facility was a residential program it was organised and completed within a week. The program would include a comprehensive case discussion with all the professionals involved. Boys Town National Research Hospital has built on those early beginnings that I observed, to have diverse and unique programs for children. There was one little touch at Boys Town that I really liked, in the residential area there were little porthole windows near the floor, the window frame was deep so the children could sit in them and be in their own little world. It was a very thoughtful touch.

It wasn't all work at Boys Town. During my stay the Nebraska speech and hearing conference was on in Lincoln. The team at Boys Town thought that the young English visitor had probably never been driven past cornfields for three hours to get to another town. They were completely correct. So they kindly took me off to the conference in Lincoln and we drove past cornfields for three hours. The conference was good but I remember the drive more.

Now I was off cross-country to San Diego. While I was here I learned more from the experts about my chosen topic of auditory electro-physiology. I learnt about the importance of getting both the recording filters and the sound parameters right. I also sampled my first Margarita, had tropical fruits for breakfast, and experienced some amazement at the sight of students going to class with sand between their toes and wearing shorts. This was certainly another first in my experience of University life. Tropical fruits weren't very common in the 70s in England either.

A highlight of my visit overall was my trip to New Orleans. My host was the famous Dr Charles Berlin at the Kresge Hearing Research Laboratory. I had been looking forward to meeting him because his research had influenced the path that I had taken in mine, although he was more senior and well regarded. In fact, the Kresge Laboratory was very important in advancing our knowledge of peripheral hearing mechanisms and of central auditory processing of sounds. I was privileged to be there. My own work had got to a point where I hoped I might have something to offer in a discussion. I had given very little thought to the fact that I was going to such a tourist destination as the French Quarter, New Orleans. I think we forget today how limited our awareness of other places was in the days before everyone is connected to the Internet.

I went to New Orleans because of Prof Berlin's academic reputation and the overlapping areas of research interest. My meetings there were fruitful, and we later collaborated on some research. Prof Berlin was also interested in how people use islands of very high frequency hearing, when they don't have much else. He was also interested in how we can use information that we record from electro-physiology to understand how important it is to get input to the brain from both ears. This fundamental understanding of how we process sound from both ears has influenced my opinion that it's important to get two hearing aids, if you have hearing loss in both ears, even if there is a better ear, in order to keep the nerve pathways actively involved. There's a lot more science now showing how important that is, but I still hear clients tell me that they have been told that one hearing aid is okay. It very rarely is. We use glasses, not a monocle; we wear two socks, and trousers with two legs. Two appropriate hearing aids are almost always the right choice. They help in the short term, so that you get more balanced input, and they help in the long term, because they keep the nerve pathways active.

I arrived in New Orleans intending to stay with a friend of a friend who I met on the way. Our meeting was to take place in the French Quarter in a hotel bar. My potential host arrived and told me that he had moved to a place out of town, after splitting up with his girlfriend. He explained that she still lived in the French Quarter and would probably be happy to have me to stay. We walked there and knocked on the door. She kindly took me in and we went on to become good friends. I was in a rather Bohemian apartment in the French quarter of New Orleans in 1979. Again I draw on my auditory memories. Kathy introduced me to Pachelbel's 'Canon', which therefore, rather oddly, makes me think of New Orleans. Through the night, I lay on the couch and listened to the sound of jazz coming in from the streets. Music was everywhere.

My host was, not only one of the Laboratory Founders, he was a well known jazz pianist too, which in an Internet era, I would have probably known. Not only did I learn a lot about hearing, I learned quite a lot about jazz too. Being in New Orleans and hosted by a jazz musician was a lot of fun, and very exotic, for the girl from England. Sadly, Dr 'Chuck' Berlin lost his home during Hurricane Katrina. I had visited him, and his team in the Communications Laboratory, at the William Pitcher

Plaza Campus, six miles from the main medical school in what he described in a monograph:

'It was magnificent squalor: all the space we could ask for (11,500 square feet), along with holes in the floor, leaks in the roof, rats, mice, and cockroaches galore, but lots of green space and plenty of parking.'

New Orleans wasn't my last stop on this generously funded fellowship. I visited the research facilities at the Naval Air Station base at Pensacola. A naval base is full of healthy young men, and hence a good place to do research on a healthy population rather than a pathological population. I was there to learn about the establishment of foundation normal data. I wore, without much thought, a pale yellow diaphanous skirt, that lead to me getting a lot more attention than I had planned.

The Naval Air Station Pensacola started as a Spanish fort, which was built in 1797. The Naval Aerospace Medical Research Laboratory was, and still is, a leader in research on the causes and cures for disorientation sickness. The research laboratory conducts research in aviation medicine and related sciences. They were able to collect normative data on very large groups, as their recruits had comprehensive medical checks. This is very valuable information, because there are few other opportunities to access such large sample sizes of information. They provided benchmarking normal data for hearing and auditory evoked potentials. This was the first time that I had thought of military personnel's contribution to medical research. It was also the occasion of my first swim on a surf beach.

One more stop on the study tour of a lifetime. This was to the American Speech and Hearing Associations, ASHA's conference in Atlanta. I formed the view, after the conference, hopefully quite wrongly that it was held for three reasons, in addition to sharing information: the first was to have as many interesting meals as possible: Food. The second was to change jobs, using the job posting board: Career. The third was to get laid: Perhaps rather uninterestingly, I stopped at Food, The music memory for this trip should have been 'Georgia on My Mind', or to be more contemporary, *Underdog*, and Atlanta Rhythm Section: 'Do it or Die'. 'Do it no matter what the people say'.

The conference was held in a venue that was extraordinary, in comparison to venues in Britain at that time. The dramatic Peachtree Centre, where the conference was held, overawed me. Most of the structures that make up the centre, including the tall tower of one of the hotels, The centre was designed by wellknown Atlanta architect, John Portman, known for his cinematic interiors, and they are distinctive partly because of the atria in a network of hotels, convention spaces and shops connected by a network of enclosed pedestrian sky bridges, well above street level. It has been criticised for cutting off the convention district from the rest of the city. Given that the hotels, once again, had interior signage saying 'don't go out', this was not a surprising side effect. The hotel spaces were gorgeous. I was captivated. I had never seen anything like it: tall towers, soaring atria, indoor sculptures and indoor pools.

When I returned, I went to an awards ceremony for the Churchill Fellows. My Churchill Fellowship award was presented to me by the late Margaret Thatcher. I gained more hearing memories, which were quite separate. This was the same day that the SAAS raided the Iranian Embassy in London to rescue the hostage after the six-day siege. More gun shots, and sadly, more deaths. Many years later, I was in Australia House on the day of Dame Margaret Thatcher's funeral. The parade passed by outside. I didn't see it, but I certainly heard it.

After America, I went to work in London, at a combination of University College, the National Hospital for Nervous Diseases, now the National Hospital for Neurology and Neurosurgery, and the Royal National Throat, Nose and Ear Hospital, known colloquially as Gray's Inn Road. I was there to develop a course in audiology for a degree in speech therapy. I was also there to run classes on a Master's degree in human communication. It was another role where I was the first incumbent. I think a history of being the first incumbent in a role, has made me very self-motivated and entrepreneurial. Once again I was very lucky with the people around me and able to draw on their expertise. Working in this environment activated my interest in clinical education.

As part of this role I worked in the auditory rehabilitation department at the Throat, Nose and Ear Hospital with a group of audiologists, psychologists, hearing therapists and medical staff in a team led by the late Dr Dafydd Stephens, known to all who knew him, as Dai. He made one of the biggest influences on my career, and under his leadership, the team developed a strongly client focused approach to auditory rehabilitation. We worked only with people who needed that service. Most people can get on with using hearing aids quite comfortably without any further help. In fact the research shows that further help is not particularly beneficial. However some people particularly people with complex problems, or people who had left getting hearing aids for too long, benefit from more instruction and support. People who needed counselling needed good counselling, and before long, the largest professional group in the team was psychologists. The experience of working in their specialist group influences me today.

We supply our hearing aids to people all over the world and they are comfortably able to set them up themselves with the tools that we give them. If they want more help we can help them with hearing aid adjustments from afar over the Internet just as if they were in our office. This is called tele-audiology. However some people prefer or need face-to-face professional support. Today, I run an audiology clinic too, for that purpose and rarely expect the consultation to last less than an hour or two. In the auditory rehabilitation unit where I worked with Dr Stephen's, our philosophy was that we would spend an hour

wanted to learn more, and I wanted to contribute more. So I started to look for the next career adventure, and it came from the direction that I would not have predicted. Now when at work, I can say,

'I come from a Land Down Under.'

CHAPTER TEN

TRANSPORTATION TO ELYSIUM FIELDS

It was time to be stretched further. I thought it would be good to work directly in diagnostic audiology: to use all this knowledge about hearing and hearing loss, but I seemed to have become too senior too quickly in Britain, so I accepted a position heading up the audiology department in a teaching hospital in Australia: the Alfred Hospital in Melbourne, to be precise. The department specialised in investigations into conditions causing hearing and balance disorders. I was to be the new head of a department that specialised in investigating the medical implications of hearing and balance disturbances.

Luckily, my transportation didn't involve a four-month ride in a wooden sailing ship. I came via the USA, on another study tour, this time funded by the multinational corporation, 3M, who then manufactured a single channel cochlear implant. The hospital in Melbourne was keen for me to start a cochlear implant program there. The study tour was great, but I soon realised that starting a cochlear implant programme in Melbourne was not a great idea for many reasons. I was a novice; I was convinced that the multichannel cochlear implant, developed by Professor Graeme Clark was the way to go, and what could I offer, when there was a very experienced team in town? The 3M single channel implant was losing ground to the multichannel implant of Nucleus, for good reason: the Nucleus device was better.

So, I arrived at the Alfred Hospital, to lead an incumbent team in diagnostic audiology. I was the imported foreign expert. The head of the team, Ann, was generous in her welcome; accepted me as her new boss, and taught me a lot. She was, and is, an outstanding clinician. The unit I worked in specialised in auditory and vestibular disorders, they are sometimes one and the same thing. Remember how the hearing and balance system are contained within one labyrinth – then it's not surprising that there are ailments that involve both hearing and balance. Some of the ailments involve the sensory detection units, in either the hearing or the balance system; some of the conditions involve the nerve pathway. The treatment of the two conditions is very different, so it's important to be able to distinguish them.

I was impressed by Melbourne. It was certainly on the music tour circuit. This was the year of the tours to Melbourne of Neil Young, INXS, Bruce Springsteen, Queen, The Magic Flute, HMS Pinafore on board Polly Woodside, and of course, the Melbourne Symphony Orchestra's numerous concerts, more hearing memories. People remember what they have heard. Sometimes people who have lost their hearing suddenly and traumatically, and then get a cochlear implant, can't really tell the difference between what they can hear and the sounds they can remember. People who get hearing aids as soon as they notice problems will enjoy a hearing aid that make sound as natural as possible because they can remember their hearing. That's why my hearing aids don't compress the sound. No one wants to listen to compressed sound really. Compression in hearing aids is based on theories of loudness that are not universally accepted. It's all to do with how the inner and outer hair cells behave, both normally and when damaged.

Not long after I arrived I was introduced to a handsome and pleasant man, who invited me sailing in his Lazy E dinghy. Despite my sailing experience, I had never gone out on a trapeze. For non-sailors, the term trapeze involves a support wire that comes from a point high on the mast to a hook on the crew member's harness, on the chest or at about waist level. The crew member stands in a braced position, feet on the side of the boat, facing the mast, clipped by a hook to the harness. One minute we were sailing, the next, I was under the water, under the sail, and firmly clipped into my harness. I'd like to say that I was quite calm. I wasn't. I panicked, and thought, 'Oh, no! I've spent all that effort coming to Australia, and now I'm going to die.' Happily, the helmsman, John, realising that I had not the faintest idea what to do, and not wanting his sail to be damaged, jumped in and rescued me. About a year later we got married. No choice really; all the best stories have the heroine marry her rescuer.

In the Alfred hospital unit we were concerned with identifying the underlying cause of a hearing or balance disorder. Disorders that affect balance can be very unpleasant, even if they are not life threatening. One of my first patients at the Alfred Hospital caused my colleagues some amusement – not at the poor young man's condition, but at the new migrants inability to handle the situation – or even understand him. The young man in question had vestibular neuronitis, or labrynthitis. This is a short, but nasty, infection of the inner ear that causes symptoms including strong dizziness. This medical problem usually gets better by itself within three or four weeks, but can persist for longer. My patient with dizziness was a sheep shearer, from a big station in the Western District, a few hundred kilometres from Melbourne. He was 24 and accustomed to being very fit. I tried to take a case history, and asked him to tell me about his medical problem. He replied in some strong Australian vernacular, indicating that he didn't feel at all well. I kind of got the gist of what he was saying, but it wasn't very specific. So I asked him to explain. He said 'I'm crook in the guts.' When I still looked a bit puzzled, he told me that he didn't much like foreigners. 'I'm not a foreigner' I thought, 'I'm an Overseas Expert.'

I enjoyed the work at Alfred Hospital, and enjoyed the challenging investigative work of diagnostic audiology. It's an experience that I would recommend to any audiologist, as it provided me with much more insight into causes and manifestations of different types of hearing and balance problems.

I served on the hospital board, many years later, and was disappointed to see that the hospital chapel had gone. I got married in the chapel – we were their second ever wedding. I know I work hard, but it raises eyebrows when I tell people that I got married at work.

I worked at the Alfred Hospital for about two years, working closely with the Ear, Nose and Throat specialists and taking on board properly the responsibility of diagnosis. Quite a lot of the work involved determining whether a hearing and balance disorder was caused by a problem in the inner ear and labyrinth, or whether it was something to do with the hearing nerve or further up the nerve pathway. Quite a lot of this work today has been made redundant by the more common use of MRI scans, which are a type of X-ray. Magnetic Resonance Imaging (MRI) is a medical imaging technique that uses a magnetic field and radio waves to take pictures of the body's interior. It can quickly demonstrate or eliminate certain conditions, such as space occupying tumours, obviating the need for lengthy audiology assessments.

One condition that was commonly suspected from the symptoms, and hence commonly investigated, was Menieres disease. Meniere's disease is a disorder of the inner ear that causes spontaneous episodes of vertigo; fluctuating hearing loss; ringing in the ear (tinnitus), and sometimes a feeling of fullness or pressure in your ear and it can affect one or both ears. It is most commonly controlled by conservative treatment, such as medication, although surgical intervention is carried out in extreme cases.

I left the Alfred Hospital to have my first child; over the next eight years I had four children. What followed was a professional period that included, casual audiology work with ENT's; considerable community work; University tutoring, and home educating my children. For some years I was involved in helping people make educational choices, and was able to leverage off some of my work with children. But perhaps the most interesting role I held was a locum position at the now demolished Mildura Base Hospital. Mildura is a regional city in North Western Victoria. I was to be there for a month, and during that time we lived in a small apartment in the hospital. If you have ever lived in an Australian country town, then you won't be surprised to hear that everyone in town quickly got to know this new family and what we did. I worked hard all day, and John took the children out and about. I loved the work, because a country audiologist has such a varied case load. I found the country people to be very resilient – accepting of problems, and of the fact that a solution was needed. I wish country people today were quicker to get on with using hearing aids. Noise induced hearing loss is endemic in rural Australia, and early action would reduce the social isolation and depression that it can lead to.

CHAPTER ELEVEN

THE CURL AT THE END OF THE ELECTRODE

A big step forward in my professional career was the day I presented myself at the Bionic Ear Institute in Melbourne and asked for a job from Professor Graeme Clark. I found the Bionic Ear Institute to be a very special place. It had a greater concentration of experts than I had ever experienced anywhere before. A researcher is accustomed to using libraries to learn more, but at the Bionic Ear Institute, it was often easier to just go and ask an expert. The world leading expert was there, on-site. This was special. This was my first full time job after some years of sharing part-time enterprises with the early years of my four children.

It was typical of Graeme to give me a chance even though I had been out of the scientific workforce for years. Of course going to the Bionic Ear Institute was exciting because the topic of cochlear implants was pretty awesome. At this time cochlear implants were often giving someone who had very little, or no, residual hearing an ability to understand speech, in good listening environments. But there was still a lot to be done, to make it work better. There is also still research going on to find out why the implant works so much better for some people than others. Although the auditory system is very orderly giving some advantages to copy implant designers, when people are deaf for a long time the hearing system reorganises itself and we don't really fully understand how. But we do know that a long period with no auditory input makes it harder to get good benefit from a cochlear implant or a hearing aid.

So, I had been working on a new curly electrode with Graeme Clark, the talented engineers at Cochlear and many surgeons around the world. The new design implant we were developing was pre-curled, that is, it went in straight, and ended up tightly curled around the central spiral of the inner ear. This meant it could be nearer to the hearing nerve, and thus more efficient. In this chapter we look at the inspirational and moving story of Jodi Harris who was an early recipient of this new device. Jodie is one of the bravest and most determined people I know. She had lost most of her hearing by the time she was five, but I think that if she had been born with only one leg she would have climbed mountains. She's an actor – today, she's an actor with a cochlear implant and mother to two beautiful children. I met her when she volunteered to be the first person to try the new generation of cochlear implants in 1998.

JODIE'S STORY AND THE SOUND OF WAVES

Jodie probably lost her hearing before she was four years old. She used hearing aids for years, and was neither signing deaf, nor easily part of the hearing world. As an oral (speaking) deaf person, she was not welcomed by the signing deaf, but she was not at home with hearing people either. I can't tell this story as well as Jodie can, so I asked her to tell it for me, and this is what she said:

'My name is Jodie Harris and I am a profoundly deaf actress with a Cochlear implant. I was diagnosed with a moderate to severe loss at the age of six but Mum was pretty sure that something was wrong well before this. My lip reading skills had already developed by this stage and the doctor repeatedly said I had a cold. I was constantly in trouble at school and home for "not doing as I was told" and mostly had no

idea why I was in trouble! For me this was normal and school was quite a scary place. When asked when did I realise I couldn't hear I responded with "When the man told me". As most kids do, I accepted what was going on around me as "normal".

It was only after a recent discussion with my mother that I realised how worried my parents were about whether they had made the right choices for me. I went to a "normal" school and my parents never allowed me any concessions that they wouldn't give to my two beautiful hearing sisters. I was the only person in my family who was deaf. I was not treated any differently and I grew up feeling "normal" or hearing. I was the one who had to make most of the adjustments in my family, and looking back there was a time as an adult I felt quite angry that my own family had made so few adjustments for me when the rest of the world was willing to. A discussion with Mum revealed that both her and Dad did this consciously as they were worried about me not having the coping mechanisms to thrive in the hearing world without their support. They never expected any less of me than they did of my sisters and I will be forever grateful and thankful that they chose to do this. Without this support and their belief in me I may not have had the courage to pursue what I always wanted to do – act. It was my escape from the world, to transform to another being and see the world from their eyes. To understand their failings, misgivings and struggles gave me some respite from my own. And to completely fool my Dad with a "performance" to my Mum's delight was half the fun!

By 13, I was profoundly deaf and blessed with lifelong friends who did not see me as any different and had high expectations for me. My school results were credible, and considering I was only picking up about a third of the information a hearing person did, I was doing really *well. But it was hard, and it was only once I received the cochlear implant 16 years later that I realised just how difficult it had been. I was in a constant state of high alert in case someone said something to me and I had a tendency to avoid using language where I was not sure of the pronunciation as there is no way I would hear the correction to fix it. It was probably about now that the rage began and if I had to create a visual impression of what happened to me inside during this time it would be one of a gradual progression to darkness and being in a box that was slowly closing in on me. I had a recurring nightmare of being very tiny and squashed between two giant boxing gloves. It was not the loss of sound that was destroying me it was the loss of the ability to be myself, my ability to be with the people I loved for any length of time without great difficulty. This loss and grief that was happening was suppressed and released with great, destructive bouts of rage directed at those closest to me. There was nothing I could do about my hearing loss, so I got on with it with no idea where this rage was coming from. I never felt sorry for myself or expected less of myself and I accepted the cold hard reality that I would have to work twice as hard to get half as far in whatever I chose to do so I might as well put the effort into what I loved and what I was good at. And, oh, for those moments in character when for a while I could escape myself and my hidden demons.'*

It is our voice that empowers us, that characterises us with others. Jodie didn't feel she had a voice. Jodie successfully got accepted into the prestigious Victorian College of the Arts, and began studying for her Bachelor of Dramatic Arts. By then she had travelled round the world, and developed many strategies to cope with her deafness.

It was six months into the course when she took the big step of getting a cochlear implant. Not only that, but she volunteered to be the first person to get the new curly electrode, she was also agreeing to hours of research with me, to work out how well it was working, and what should be done next. Meanwhile, Jodie tells of her actor training and how she found her voice.

'And so commenced my acting training and three years intensive investigation of my voice under the expert guidance of Geraldine Cook who was a Senior Lecturer at VCA. The best way I can describe my voice before this investigation is as being high, thin, lacking vibration and unconnected to breath. There is no way I could make it travel to the back of a theatre and even those in the first row would have struggled. I could not make myself heard in a group conversation and being unaware that this was the problem thought that no one was interested in what I had to say. I felt small, insignificant and very much like a mouse! I knew that this wasn't me but I couldn't be me. I had lost myself.'

So, at a critical time in her career, she decided to get a cochlear implant, and volunteered to be the recipient of a new device. She was studying full time, working part time and giving many hours a week as a cochlear implant (bionic ear) research volunteer for the benefit of others. We were a team.

Many times she would study all night, in order to be available in the early morning to carry out her research role, before going in to college. But more exciting things were to come. Jodie realised that her acting training was helping her adjust to her new hearing experience, and to help her find her new voice.

Cochlear Ltd won the Australian Design Award for the new electrode design in 2000, and invited both Jodie and me to the ceremony. Jodie was unexpectedly summoned to the stage to speak her words: 'In giving Cochlear this award, you should be proud of yourselves. This device hasn't just given me back my hearing. It's given me back my life.' There wasn't a dry eye in the theatre. When Jodie finished her degree, and was looking for acting work, she still found time to help others. She continued on the path of a personal and professional investigation of 'hearing and being heard', both of which she had found necessary to be fully connected to the hearing community. Jodie told me about her vision:

'Geraldine and I discovered so much about my voice. At the end of VCA I do not believe I had integrated my voice with my acting fully but I had come a long way and we both had much that we wanted to share with other's in my situation. Not only did I feel I had my hearing back, I also had a voice in the community now and people listened to me. I was empowered and had become part of the wider community again. I have lived two completely different lives. Before and after and it literally happened overnight. It was huge and emotional, exciting and challenging, an absolute roller coaster ride.'

I gave Jodie a desk to use for her project and a part time job as my personal assistant, a role she performed spectacularly well. Jodie used this launch platform to successfully raise grant money for a research program in vocal empowerment: a program designed to understand the effect of how actor vocal training could help young people with cochlear implants. This was a project where arts and medicine collided. Jodie still found time to work for me in an international business, that had spun out of cochlear implant work where we were developing technologies for hearing aid companies, it was plain to me that Jodie's challenges gave her a focus that was immensely valuable to an early stage company on a tight budget.

The Vocal Empowerment study comprised seven adolescents who had received cochlear implants, and who relied on oral communication. Her studies showed that the program led to: a significant reduction in stress; increased confidence in using their voices in public spaces; a strengthening of personal identity for the young people; significantly better voice pitch control; better expressivity (through use of wider pitch span) and a significant decrease in speaking rate. The work lead to several publications and presentations, so that many more people could be helped by this work.

Jodie is still involved in the ongoing training and research in the 'Let it Out!' program. The team is developing online training modules teaching actor vocal training to people with hearing difficulties. She currently runs this program at Methodist Ladies College with their hearing impaired unit.

'Geraldine and I have passed this work on successfully to a group of young people and they are doing magnificently. Maybe they would have achieved everything they have without the program we developed with and for them but I like to think we can take a little credit! This work led to The Sound of Waves, originally a research outcome from my work with Geraldine and this group. It gave me the opportunity to push the boundaries of my voice in performance. It is a fairy tale and like the best fairy tales has truth as its essence. It maps the emotional landscape and turmoil, the ups and downs in a much more effective way than I do in this letter to you. It traces the experience of a little girl who had no idea things were not quite right in her world, to a rage ridden monster, to post operation/post vocal investigation confusion and the struggle to work it all out, to this very day, when yes, like most of us, I am still trying to work it all out!

'I love it because it makes people laugh, it touches their soul and it

makes me aware that what I have experienced – loss, grief, isolation,
despair, depression, hope, joy, laughter – is universal. This is not only
my story. This show makes me feel less alone because people say to
me "I know what you mean", "I have been where you have been", "I
am watching my mum, dad, brother, sister, friend go through this" and
mostly, "You need to share this story with more people". It has the
power that theatre can have to connect people to each other and tell
them a story that changes them in some way.'

In *The Sound of Waves*, Jodie played six characters, it is an allegorical tale of the journey into the isolation of deafness and the return to communication, as she found her voice.

Jodie was also involved in the creative development of *The Cat Lady of Bexley*, for the Australian Theatre of the Deaf in Sydney. In 2008 she had a major role in a short film, and took part in radio plays, including for ABC Radio.

Jodie is an extraordinary person, who has achieved so much against a background of deafness, but she always finds time to help others overcome the challenge of deafness and isolation. Jodie and I have a special bond that I struggle to describe. I suppose it comes from being together as research partners and friends through this incredibly critical period of her life. Neither of us feels it's necessary to find the words.

When I saw *The Sound of Waves,* shown to only a small invited audience, I found the impact enormous, this is how I came to add producer to my resume. I knew I had to give Jodie the opportunity to develop this further and take it to the world. I'm not wealthy, but I put up all I can find so that the play goes on. So has Peter, my business partner, and somehow I'm finding the rest. In October 2014, *The Sound of Waves,* played to the Melbourne public, which was funded by philanthropy. After a lifetime working to help reduce the problems of hearing loss, and a lifetime of community work, trying to raise awareness of hearing difficulties, I have embarked on an amazing new venture with Jodie. *The Sound of Waves* is the story of Shelly, a 'double tailed mermaid', part human and part fish, who becomes 'more and more fish every day'. She escapes into a world under the sea where she finds refuge from life on land, which is becoming more unbearable as time goes on, until one day she finds herself at the bottom of the ocean. There, she is under immense pressure, and this increases with the arrival of an Anglerfish. This pushes her to the surface and she learns to walk on land again. It is a whimsical, emotionally compelling one woman show written by Gareth Ellis, directed by Naomi Edwards and created and performed by the profoundly deaf, Jodie Harris. It's a metaphorical autobiography of Jodie's real life experience. We are doing this because we know that many people will be moved by this tale, but many people will relate to the tale, identifying their own experiences of isolation, grief, loneliness, loss, depression, achievement, hope and possibility. The first night of the show nearly brought me to tears. Theatre can tell a story so much more strongly than mere words. When I met Jodie, I was leading the research team, for the new curly electrode, which was to be hers. My strongest picture of Jodie is captured by the image of her just before her cochlear implant operation. The science, engineering and medical teams had worked for months to be sure that we had the best shot at success, and that the new electrode was safe to implant into people. Safe means that it wouldn't damage the very delicate structures of the inner ear, or worse. It's still a bit nerve wracking, though, to see a young women with a little bit of hearing that she relied on, and a career goal of being an actor, go into surgery to get a new generation, and hence untried, cochlear implant. It seems I let my anxiety show, and Jodie was all care for me, even as she went under the sedation for anaesthetic. She looked at me, took my hand

and said, 'Don't worry Elaine.' I wasn't the one on the hospital trolley. I wasn't the one whose remaining bit of hearing was at stake.

Jodie's implant was, and is, successful. I've seen her play Puck, in *A Midsummer Night's Dream,* with cunning hair styling so it wasn't visible, and didn't fall off. The new design implant was successful, and went on to be the basis of many more improvements. Jodie devoted hours and hours of time listening to sounds with me, so that we could learn more about why it was working. In other words, she became a research volunteer and donated many hours for the sole reason that it would help other people hear even better with their cochlear implant in the future. We also became good friends, with something of a special bond due to our path as partners in her hearing.

My part of the cochlear implant story was modest, but meant very long hours, a lot of time away from my family, and the chance to work with some wonderful, clever and determined people all around the world. My special research role was early work on the new curled electrode, which eventually led to the new generation of Cochlear implants that Jodie trialled. There was a whole phase of research before Jodie and indeed before I became involved, I did a lot of research work with three special volunteers who elected to try an early iteration of the device. To work with these three volunteers was extensive and intensive, as a special bond builds up between the researchers and the volunteers, which derives from very long hours of collaborative listening work. Volunteers first have made the bold step to agree to be a guinea pig with a new device and then they commit to weekly sessions or more to listen to sounds for hours at a time to test and find out how well the device is working. The work to improve and understand the Cochlear implant and the hearing mechanism is part of a discipline called psychophysics. This is a general term to describe the relationship between physical stimuli and the sensations and perceptions they cause. So a hearing test is a type of psychophysical task; in that case we might call it psychoacoustics. However, we use predominantly electrical stimuli in cochlear implant research, so we use the more general term of psychophysics.

One of my three volunteers with the earlier version of a pre-curved electrode, was Joanna and we had much in common. We were similar in age and both had four young children about the same age. Her life history however, was very different to mine. She had no memory of ever having had hearing which wasn't a particularly auspicious start to her future with a cochlear implant, experimental or otherwise when the hearing system has not been used for a long time, if ever, then the likelihood of success with a cochlear implant is markedly reduced. When I first started working with Joanna she wasn't terribly confident, but she was extremely bright and became quite interested in the research itself and the use of the computer test protocols. It's quite normal in psychophysics to present the test stimuli, and then to ask the volunteer to make judgements and tell the researcher (me), what they had heard. Joanna wanted to take over the computer because that would be more direct for her, and more efficient than telling me what she was hearing. She wanted to take control and adjust the test stimuli herself. Joanna's need to take control sowed seeds in my mind. It's sensible for people to adjust their own hearing aids. For years, hearing aid companies have been making it so complicated to set up hearing aids, that you had to pay an expert to set them up for you. In later years, I was able to put this together, to supply hearing aids people set up themselves, so that they too can 'take control' of their hearing aids. Joanna had a very busy life: she was studying part time while working part time and she was the main carer for her children. Sometimes when she came in, she was really tired and her tolerance and interpretation of sound was influenced by this. Fatigue, attention and listening are all connected. Judgements of noise, loudness, what we like to hear, and what we find annoying is influenced by our state of mind.

I am no longer in touch with Joanna. However her contribution to cochlear implant and hearing aid research was much bigger than she could have known. For her part, gaining some extra auditory information and taking part in the research paper must have given her a confidence to take on new challenges that she may not have otherwise done.

I was leading a team and coordinating the work of some very bright people, enabling them to work well together to solve problems. I had discovered I was quite an effective team leader. I realised that the team leader didn't have to be the most senior or the cleverest member of the team. I have used these skills many times since and written articles on team leading, as the team went through the classic stages of Forming, Storming, Performing and Ending. I hadn't read the management books then, so I didn't realise that I was working to the text, but I pulled the team together and found ways of making it work effectively. We achieved a terrific outcome, and then we were not really needed anymore. The work had moved inside Cochlear Ltd and they were building their own team, that didn't rely on external collaborators. This was a great result. The overall research involved a lot of people around the world. My memories of surgical research mingle with pictures of testing the hearing of deaf children in Southern Germany, whilst the snow fell thickly outside – in itself an unusual experience for an Australian scientist.

The pre-curved electrode experience was a personal lesson in overcoming obstacles. I'm reminded again of my boss and helmsman Ross Coles, calling out to me 'It's not "I can't", it's "How".' The next stages of the research called for a lot of lateral thinking and innovation. The goal was to get an electrode that would curl tightly around the spiral of the cochlear, because the nerves are in that spiral, the nearer you are to the nerve, the less current is needed. This doesn't sound so hard, but unfortunately, to get the electrode into place, the procedure is such that it has to go down a straight tunnel about one and a half centimetres long. This is the tunnel in the bone of the skull which leads to the inner ear. A gifted young engineer at Cochlear Ltd. came up with the design of the new electrode, it had to go through rigorous safety testing. The safety testing took two forms. One was a very traditional biomedical approach, which was to insert electrodes into the cochlea in temporal bones and evaluate the safety and efficacy of the insertion. The goal was to not damage the structures in the ear. The second, I introduced, and was an engineering risk assessment. We had to do lots of different things to show that the new electrode would do what it was supposed to do, and wouldn't do irreversible harm, to the delicate inner ear structures. This is a story that can be told in slightly different ways for any medical device that will be implanted in the body. The engineers and inventors want to do good and they mustn't do harm.

There wasn't an easy path to some of the measures we wanted to do. We had to show, in temporal bones, that the electrode was easy to go in, and would sit in the right place, the electrode is very small. A temporal bone is a section of the skull that includes the ear. People donate temporal bones to research, in a similar manner to choosing to donate other body parts.

We had to do lots of things that hadn't been invented, so I had to find people who could develop solutions. We needed to make a video X-ray of the electrode going into a temporal bone. Preliminary research showed that micro-video fluoroscopy, as it is known, would be suitable, but it was not readily available. So we worked with a local company, XRT, to set up a custom imaging set up. The system was set up on an industrial inspection machine, containing a narrow beam X-ray tube, and the potential for video recording. This was a terrific collaboration between the Department of Otolaryngology staff, from the University of Melbourne, in particular, Dr Xu, and a local company. It was incredibly important that the cochlear implant electrode was easy to insert and caused minimal damage. We also needed to look at something that was very small. Fortunately I was, as has often happened, working with some very clever people, and Dr Jin Xu, currently of the Bionics Institute, worked with me to source equipment so that she could develop special X-ray techniques, that were also safe for the researchers. This work was the precursor to the development of a more sophisticated imaging lab, but that was a few years down the track, and after I had moved on. We worked a lot with XRT, which was founded in the late 90s to commercialise unique X-ray phase contrast imaging technology originally developed by the Commonwealth Scientific and Industrial Research Organisation (CSIRO) in Melbourne. The CSIRO group continues to be active in this field and XRT enjoys a close relationship with them. Jin did a lot with phase contrast, the phase contrast microscope is a vital instrument in biological and medical research when dealing with transparent and colourless components in a cell, dyeing is an alternative but at the same time stops all processes in it. The phase contrast microscope has made it possible to study living cells, and cell division is an example of a process that has been examined in detail with it. The phase contrast microscope was awarded with the Nobel Prize in Physics, 1953.

So, I found a group of people in Melbourne who were game to make one: XRT, with Dr. Xu's help. We needed to insert the electrode into the cochlea in temporal bones of deceased people. The surgeons would take several cochleas, and implant the electrodes. The trouble is the cochlea is a closed structure and you can't tell from the outside as to whether you have inserted the electrode without damaging any of the delicate structures of the inner ear. The X-ray technique gave some information, but we wanted more. After the insertion, the temporal bone, containing the cochlea and the electrode, were immersed in resin. The resin we used was a viscous liquid, and set hard. This preserved the temporal bone, the cochlea and the electrode and captured a moment in time. We wanted to slice this structure thinly, so that we could see how well the electrode sat in the cochlea, and whether any damage had been caused. This sounds easy. The trouble is, the electrode is hard and tough, and the rest of the structure is very brittle. We didn't know how to do the slicing, but the dental researchers did. So they did the slicing. I had lots of visits to the Dental school in Melbourne. I love this story. It's one where today we might say 'finding enabling technology', to me it says, learn to describe the problem you have, and look for someone to solve it. I never tell people how to solve the problem. I just try and describe the outcome I need, and leave it to the experts.

All this time, our safety studies were following the typical medical safety path; the goal was to have a high proportion of good results. I wanted to introduce the second risk analysis technique. My husband John's background is in engineering risk so he coached me in the techniques of engineering risk assessment, and then arranged for his expert colleagues to facilitate workshops for me. The result of this is that we identified potential hazards that we were able to avoid because of this work. I'm proud of this work because it saved lives. At least one other company in the cochlear implant field may not have gone through this approach and didn't avoid the problem that we managed to. Oddly enough in the late 90s this level of risk analysis was not routinely applied in the development of implant devises.

Today this risk engineering approach is commonplace. At our first risk workshop, one of the research surgeons said he thought the biggest risk of this procedure would be if any air was trapped in the cochlea, the patient could die from an infection that would quickly travel into the brain, so the electrode must have a design that minimised that risk. Initially, the group reaction was sceptical. We were developing a cochlear implant electrode. How was anyone going to die? But the medical debate continued. If you are familiar with evaluation of risk, you will know that it involves looking at how likely a scenario is, and what the consequences are if it happens. Clearly death is pretty serious, so the team firmly endorsed minimising this risk in the design and the insertion technique.

I presented this work at a conference, a year or two later. It wasn't a presentation highlight for me. Instead it was a good example of trying to be a female engineer giving a talk amongst male medicos. I was first on straight after lunch, but the session started late. The chair person started to ring his bell for 'Time's up', a few minutes into my talk. At that point, I accidentally dropped my notes for my talk, I had some pages missing, and those pages were lying on the floor between the lectern, where I was standing, and my seat. That was the last time I have ever used notes for a talk or presentation. I was quite upset, because I like to do things well, and this was going badly wrong. I then realised that penetrating the conference circuit of male medicos was tough. A lesson learned, and not one to be forgotten. Back to Melbourne, back to reality.

As in all stages of my career, I met some fantastic people. An enterprising researcher from the University of Antwerp, Peter Deman, came to visit us in Melbourne, at the Bionic Ear Institute to learn more about cochlear implant safety studies. He was developing an electrode along a very different path, but we were collaborating on the safety measures and not the technology per se. He was as earnest and as much of a workaholic as me, which was thoroughly demonstrated when my family took him for a walk and a picnic to one of my favourite places, Cape Schanck in Victoria. We shared the beach gear and picnic to carry on the several kilometre walk to the beach. Peter's bag was heavy. When we got to the beach, he produced a pile of books and papers for discussion, a man after my own heart! It's a pity the event pre dated the iPad! Peter Deman went back to Belgium, and soon published a most interesting PhD thesis.

By the mid-1980s there were sufficient stories of astonishing success that people started to believe a device had finally been invented that gave extraordinarily good hearing and communication ability to people who had been profoundly deaf. Newspaper articles in many countries had carried stories of greatly improved lives from the recipients of cochlear implants. But as in many areas of medical science, the path to the successes of today was far from easy. In truth, the results were promising enough that it was worth the time, determination and fight of many scientists, engineers, clinicians and philanthropists.

At that time, I was working in England, in the NHS, and at University College. I couldn't see how this new technology could fit into the future health economics of Britain. I was very wrong. Today, the cochlear implant is so much better than most of us could have dreamt of, and I'm proud to have played a little part in that progress. Perhaps I was most proud the day I watched Jodie enjoy her carefully chosen wedding music – it is always emotional at a wedding – but seeing a profoundly deaf young woman enjoying her wedding music was extraordinary, and it was one of the happiest moments of my career.

Several research groups around the world pushed hard during the 1970s to make the dream of electrical stimulation of the cochlea a reality. In 1957, in Paris, a brave surgeon, Charles Eyries, implanted an electrode, of a type he used in his physiological research on hearing, into the cochlear of a patient, where he was already carrying out radical ear surgery. The outcome was not particularly successful, but gave him the conviction that there was promise in pursuing electrical stimulation of the cochlear as a treatment for cochlear deafness. The following years of research on three continents are filled with personal stories of endeavour, personality clashes and scientific differences, the involvement of industry, financing difficulties, and bravery from early participants in the field. One of the pioneers was Graeme Clark, who I hold in high esteem. Graeme was a determined entrepreneur and was good at hiring people to solve problems. He was also persistent in raising money. He is much lauded for his pioneering medical innovation, but the part of his story that intrigues me is his determination as an entrepreneur and his ability to find the right people. The result of his work is not just the Australian multichannel cochlear implant but also a longstanding contribution of a culture of research in hearing and high standards of medical device safety.

I came to Australia on a cochlear implant ticket. I came to lead advanced methods of hearing assessment at Melbourne's leading teaching hospital, The Alfred. I was also intending to launch the cochlear implant program there – supported by 3M, who were then manufacturing a single channel cochlear implant that had been developed at the American House Ear Institute. Coming from England, I was only marginally aware of Cochlear Nucleus; the relative advantages of the two systems was still under debate, and I didn't realise that it was like bringing coal to Newcastle. The superiority of the Australian Nucleus system soon became clear to me, and anyway, I didn't have the temerity to work with patients when there was so much experience so near.

Dr House's work was, however, important in the overall story. The House Ear Institute was named after Howard House, William's brother, in 1946. William was a cochlear implant and ear surgery pioneer, widely known as Dr Bill. He was one of the leaders in the path to developing practical cochlear implants. William House died in 2013, at the age of 89. The story goes that Dr House learned about the French work on cochlear implants from a newspaper article, which had been given to him by one of his patients. Dr House was sufficiently inspired by this outcome that he set to work, with an innovative engineer called Jack Urban, to develop an auditory electric stimulation system himself. House's crucial contribution to the project was to develop the surgical pathway needed, and lead to a patient being implanted in the late 1960s. The House team started off with a system of five electrodes spaced over a distance of about 20 mm and this could be inserted to various points around the cochlea. The five individual electrodes had their ends exposed, the researchers found that their first patient heard a different tone according to which electrode was stimulated.

Their work came to a halt due to the lack of suitable enabling technologies and in particular the lack of biocompatible materials. When the work resumed the decision was made to use a single electrode, which they felt had some advantages and few disadvantages. Their work led to the first FDA approved cochlear implant, which was taken to market by 3M in 1984. 3M eventually pulled out, of the cochlear implant market though because, and I quote Dr. House, 'because the Australian device came on so well.' Nucleus, as the Australian company was then known, took over the care of the 3M cochlear implant patients. Jack Urban, sadly, died in 1985, and a great surgical/engineering partnership was lost. However research in California continued. Blair Simmons at Stamford, Robin Michelson at UCSF, and Dr House's former cochlear implant study group, which was important in building a network of exchange and development of ideas.

Meanwhile, things were moving along in Australia. The story of the development of the Australian cochlear implant is an inspiring one and a story that has been told in several different books already. I believe it's a story of vision, medical science, persistence, team leadership and collaboration between scientists and entrepreneurs. In particular it is a story of Graeme Clark and his leadership of teams of engineers and scientists, and his partnership with innovative engineers, where names like Jim Patrick and Joe Tong have become legend to subsequent generations of researchers. It is also a story of an amazing entrepreneur, Paul Trainor who was the visionary owner of the Nucleus group that would ultimately bring the Nucleus multichannel cochlear implant to the market. Research and development of medical devices in Australia, as in the other research groups around the world, owes much to the brave and generous volunteers who are prepared to try experimental devices and to continue as part of research teams to evaluate how well they are working. The research volunteers that I have met in my work in cochlear implant research have been more than inspiring. They have been my heroes. I think much of their selfless persistence comes from knowing the despair that deafness can bring, and a goal to help other people in the journey back to hearing.

Paul Trainor was the owner of the Nucleus group, which included Telectronics, an Australian heart pacemaker firm. He was generous in his directing the team of expert bio-engineers that would ultimately bring the Nucleus multi-channel cochlear implant to the commercial market. My piece was very small, but I have another tale that shows even very small parts can change lives.

CHAPTER TWELVE

Just like winning the lottery...

My parents lived in England and my father had become quite ill so I made a number of trips to spend time with them. This involved quite a lot of train travel when I got to England. One trip led to a conversation with a woman who told me her worries about what do with her deaf son. I shared the knowledge I had, as anyone would, and did my best to help. We didn't exchange cards; the Internet was not omnipresent, and we lost touch. Some years later she contacted me and has shared this story, which I'm sharing with you because you never know when your one brick in the wall is an important brick:

This is Hughan's mother's story:

'Meeting Dr Elaine Saunders on the train in 1989 between London Paddington station and Exeter station in England, was just like winning the lottery for us and has had a huge impact on our lives!

'We had boarded the train on 22 December at four o'clock in the afternoon. The train was packed with Christmas shoppers and we asked this Lady if she minded if we sat with her. She explained that she had travelled from Australia and was on her way to visit her mother in Exeter.

'We were on holiday from Botswana visiting family in England and

we had taken the opportunity to see an Ear, Nose and Throat Specialist and an Audiologist in Harley Street that day with our son Hughan who was diagnosed profoundly deaf at 14 months old; at the time he was 16 months old. We were aware Hughan could not hear us at 9 months old, and it had taken five months to get his diagnosis and be given his first hearing aids. We had desperately been searching for answers on how to deal with his deafness and how we should be teaching him his communication skills in the future.

'On the train we explained to her why we had been to London and about Hughan's hearing loss. We couldn't believe it when the Lady told us she had been to University with the Audiologist we had seen earlier in the day, and started explaining that she was studying deafness and all about a device called the "Cochlear Implant". It was still in the early stages of being developed and she gave us some details about how the equipment worked and that the Australian device was ahead in technology at the time. This gave us huge hope for how we could maybe help Hughan in the future.

'When Hughan turned three years old he was unable to hear most speech sounds using his powerful hearing aids, so we had to choose between a signing programme or the Cochlear Implant. Because of the information that we had been told that day on the train in 1989, we didn't hesitate with the idea of Hughan having the Cochlear Implant, especially if it was the Australian device. He was the 10th child to receive the Cochlear Implant in Cape Town in 1992. England had not started giving children the Cochlear Implant yet.

'Since 1989 we had lost contact with the Lady we met on the train, after having moved from Botswana to Cape Town (so Hughan could be taught to use his Cochlear Implant equipment) and then to Zimbabwe in

1994 before moving on to England in 1997.

'In October 2011, I came across a packet with our train tickets and a small piece of paper with the name Dr Elaine Saunders and an Australian address on it. I decided to Google the name "Dr Elaine Saunders" and couldn't believe it when I found all the information about the incredible work she has done since we had met her on the train in 1989. After finding her email address, I was able to email her to ask her if she was the person we had met that day on the train, and she was!

'It has been truly wonderful being able to say "Thank you" to Dr Elaine Saunders for all the information she gave us that day on the train. The Cochlear Implant has had a huge impact on our son's life. Hughan, now 25, drives and owns his own car and he works full time servicing caravans. He has recently travelled by himself to visit family in South Africa. He is now even able to hold a normal conversation on a telephone. Strangers assume that he has normal hearing!

'Words can't express how thankful we are for having met Dr Elaine Saunders all those years ago. Just like winning the lottery!'

Everything we do can be like one small drop in the ocean, just one more brick in the wall. I am so happy I helped, and hope that I am always vigilant to opportunities.

DAD'S ADVICE IN HEARING LOSS

My Dad said: 'It does not pay to keep your hearing aid a secret – rather the reverse in fact.' I find this fascinating, since the history of hearing aid development has been a drive to make hearing aids less visible for the wearer. Even today, people will seek out invisible hearing aids, without asking about their quality and performance.

It is important for people who have hearing aids to watch the face of the person speaking. Actually it's important for everyone to listen with their eyes. Unless you have super human hearing, you rely on your eyes to hear when hearing conditions are poor. We have four engines for hearing, two eyes and two ears. With hearing aids with automatic (adaptive) directional microphones, then turning your head (the beam of the microphones) towards the person speaking, will give a person, better than normal hearing in many situations of background noise. The combination of the eyes and the automatic adaptive directional microphones will put you into a different class of hearers and listeners, although the advantage is reduced in reverberant rooms.

Reverberation occurs in large rooms, particularly with reflective surfaces. Sound gets reflected until surrounding objects eventually absorbs it. Reflected sounds are delayed relative to the original sound and come from multiple different directions. This disturbs the timing and localisation cues that are important for listening in noise. It makes hearing especially difficult for hearing aid users, as people with hearing loss often have poor ability to code timing differences in sound (temporal cues). The time for reverberation to completely die away depends upon how loud the sound was to begin with, and the characteristics of the room. Reverberation is a worse problem in large rooms with high ceilings and glass or unfurnished wall surfaces. Reverberation causes a greater challenge to elderly listeners than young people.

My father didn't get to be elderly, but he realised the additional burden for a hearing aid user of a reverberant room. His advice was:

'Watch the speaker, it is important that the speakers face, and especially the mouth, should actually be in view and adequately lit – not for instance with his or her back to the window. The job of interpreting conversation is that much more difficult if the talkers head is turned away.'

Dad was of course spot on. Some speech sounds are easier to read on the lips than others. Mostly, it is consonants that are easier to see on lips. This is convenient, as with age related deafness, it's the high frequencies that deteriorate first, but there is an effect on children too – hearing loss in children, where only one ear or only some frequencies, are damaged, can sometimes remain undetected as an intelligent child can make up for the hearing loss by excellent use of vision and context.

Any book or advice on active listening will advise you to look at the speaker. Most people will notice when the sound track and the visual in a film are out of time with each other. It's an uncomfortable experience, and most people pick up the problem straight away, because their hearing and lip-reading signals don't match up. Looking is such an important part of hearing; my father went on to say:

'For the same reason, you may well experience difficulty in interpreting speech on the radio. Television is rather easier, particularly the "formal" programmes such as the News in which the speakers face in sharply in focus.'

My father wrote these words more than twenty years ago. Today television style is more casual, and subtle, and a variety of regional accents occur, so I'm not sure that this is really true anymore – certainly, most of my clients tell me about problems with hearing television. I think he knew and appreciated the path that hearing aids had come. Let's take a brief look at the history, and see what happens next.

CHAPTER THIRTEEN

FROM THEN TO NOW – THE CHANGING LOOK AND SOUND OF HEARING AIDS

Not so long ago, the sounds of silence might have been better than the sound through most hearing aids. For many hundreds of years, variants of acoustic hearing aids, or ear trumpets were used well into the 20th century. Ear trumpets were available from the NHS in Britain from 1948 to 1976. Beethoven's career involved hearing, so it's not surprising that he was proactive in seeking solutions for deafness. The nature of Beethoven's hearing loss was that he managed better with music than speech. He also, at one point, used a resonant device, in order to better 'feel' the piano. He probably used both hearing and vibration as time went on, with the emphasis changing. But that's me speculating. In 1813 he had Johann Nepomuk Mälzel, an inventor of mechanical devices, produce several ear trumpets, which he called hearing machines, although he didn't find the results very satisfying. Mälzel developed a number of differently shaped ear trumpets for the composer, which partly were to be attached to the head with a metal circlet, as he had to have a 'hands free device' to play the piano. Four of those hearing aids can be seen today in the Beethoven-Haus in Bonn.

Professor Ruth Bentler, who works at the University of Iowa, published some research that she had carried out, in the mid 1990s, where she examined the impact of the changes in hearing aid technology over the years. She asked twenty volunteers to sit through a number of different types of hearing tests, using hearing aids that were representative of a particular era of technology. In one of the tests, the volunteers listened to sentences in background noise, and the experimenter measured how many words the listener identified correctly. At sound levels of about the level of a human shout, the listeners did just as well with the most up to date hearing aid, no hearing aid or a speaking tube (a type of ear trumpet). Some of the tests showed better improvement over the stages of technology, and there were designs that were less obtrusive and obvious than the ear trumpets. Progress was being made, but in the area that engineers thought mattered most, you might as well stick to the speaking tube at that time. They were very easy to maintain. In 1882, James Campbell, who was a professor in the Homeopathic Medical College of Missouri, wrote:

'The deaf are, as a rule, very sensitive over their infirmity, and hence dislike any instrument which is conspicuous, or makes this condition more apparent; for this reason many other devices have been invented, which seek to conceal this fact.'

Appearance would continue to dominate hearing aid use, and still does today. Speaking tubes and ear trumpets are both known as types of acoustic hearing aids, as distinct from electronic hearing aids that need a power source. An ear trumpet has a sound collection component and an earpiece tailored to go into the ear canal. They were easy to hold in one hand, and sometimes very decorative. The ear trumpet is a very logical invention. Most people instinctively use a cupped hand when they need a little extra help to hear. There are descriptions of using a cupped hand, and later using a 'hands free' version, which were small parchment cups behind the ears. The ear trumpet is a small, but significant step forward from a cupped hand. The general theory behind ear trumpets is to capture more sound and to provide some directionality towards the wanted sounds, while at the same time sheltering the ear from the unwanted background sounds. This is not much different from what modern digital hearing aids attempt to do electronically. We have evidence of nature's use of ear trumpets, bats that nest inside curled leaves get amplification help from the shape to transmit their messages to other bats.

Ear trumpets are most effective when used close up with the person speaking directly into the opening. But, when an ear trumpet is used to hear sounds at a distance, they have the same problem as any other hearing aid – they are collecting sound more indiscriminately, and will have other unwanted sounds mixed in with the target sound.

Speaking tubes are actually a bit different. They are made up of both a speaking end, for the speaker, connected by a tube to an earpiece for the listener. The sound is therefore direct transmission. This is a bit like a hearing aid with a remote pick up microphone today. Many children will have made a homemade version of the speaking tube, from bedroom to bedroom, or tree house to ground. One of the earliest descriptions of a speaking tube was thought to have existed as an early surveillance device, in 400BC in a mountain in Sicily. In reality, this had a somewhat different goal than, say, hearing a conversation across the dining table. It consisted of a long tube designed to convey the sound from the dungeon in the foot of the mountain to the, what was known as The Monitoring Room, at the summit. It's thought that its purpose was to eavesdrop on the prisoners, to detect any plotting, in particular escape plans that might have been going on.

The famous 'Hawksley Catalogue of Oto-acoustical Instruments to aid the Deaf', published in 1883, lists an extraordinary collection of assistive hearing devices. I particularly like the Staniland of Water Canteen, this was seen primarily as a tabletop device, although it's not hard to imagine the possible user, who, legend says, was a deafened African rubber planter who desired a portable, yet camouflaged, hearing device that could be used while on horseback supervising the workers on his plantation. A curious speciality of an acoustic chair, effectively based on speaking tube technology, was developed in the early 19th century.

British aurist and oculist John Harrison Curtis, who in 1816, established the first hospital devoted to ear diseases, known as the Royal Dispensary for Diseases of the Ear, developed one of the first Acoustic Chairs. Curtis was a lecturer in the anatomy, physiology and pathology of the ear and the eye. The sixth edition of his book, *A Treatise on the Physiology and Pathology of the Ear*, published in 1836, included a description of his Acoustic Chair:

'My Acoustic Chair is so constructed, that, by means of additional tubes, &c., the person seated in it may hear distinctly, while sitting perfectly at ease, whatever transpires in any apartment from which the pipes are carried to the chair; being an improved application of the principles of the speaking pipes now in general use. This invention is further valuable, and superior to all other similar contrivances, as it requires no trouble or skill in the use of it; and is so perfectly simple in its application, that a child may employ it with as much facility, and as effectually, as an adult. It is, moreover, a very comfortable and elegant piece of furniture. This chair is the size of a large library one, and has a high back, to which are affixed two barrels for sound, so constructed as not to appear unsightly, and at the extremity of each barrel is a perforated plate, which collects sound into a paraboloid vase from any part of the room. The instrument thus contrived gathers sound, and impresses it more sensibly by giving to it a small quantity of air. The convex end of the vase serves to reflect the voice, and renders it more distinct. Further, the air enclosed in the tube being also excited by the voice, communicates its action to the ear, which thus receives a stronger

impression from the articulated voice, or indeed any other sound.
What first induced me to invent this chair was the fatigue I sometimes
experienced in talking to deaf persons.'

Frederick Rein was another instrument manufacturer interested in acoustic devices. He established commercial production of ear trumpets in London, in 1800. He also sold speaking tubes, which helped amplify sounds. However, the devices were generally too bulky to be popular. Smaller, hand-held ear trumpets became more commonly used. He too became interested in the design of an acoustic chair and his big opportunity came when he was commissioned to design a special acoustic chair for the ailing King John II of Portugal. As an early custom designed hearing aid, which has become a legend, the throne was designed with ornately carved arms that looked like the open mouths of lions. The holes acted as the receiving area for the acoustics, which were transmitted to the back of the throne via a speaking tube, and then on into the king's ear.

Rein went on to pioneer many notable designs, including his 'acoustic headbands', where the hearing aid device was concealed within the hair or headgear. The headbands were made in a variety of shapes that incorporated sound collectors near the ear that would amplify the acoustics. Just as today, people would trade good sound quality over appearance. Perhaps a leader in this area, and one of my favourites, was the star item made by FC Rein's, called the 'Floral Aurolese Phones'. The Aurolese phones were made in various different shapes, including shells and fluted funnels resembling open flowers, as the name suggests. They were painted delicate colours, and had an earpiece and sound collector for each ear.

By the end of the 19th century, hearing aids, that are acoustic hearing aids, were serious business. Hawkley's again had time to make some observations, though:

'A deaf person is always more or less a tax upon the kindness and forbearance of friends. It becomes a duty, therefore, to use any aid which will improve the hearing and the enjoyment of the utterances of others without any murmuring about its size or appearance.'

But also a word of advice that we would do well to attend to today:

'The deaf also have a just complaint against many of their friends and public speakers, who render their affliction apparently greater by an indistinct and mumbling utterances.'

Modern electronic, or electro-acoustic hearing aids pick up sound at the microphone and converts the sounds into electrical signals. The signals are sent on to the amplifier, where the electrical signals are amplified and processed. The electrical signals are then converted back into sound at the little loud speaker.

The early powered hearing aids used a carbon membrane to vary the electrical battery voltage, to amplify the sound. The carbon membrane was essentially a carbon microphone acting as an amplifier. Much development in hearing aid technology progressed because of developments in phone technology and the rapidly emerging industry of telecommunications. The carbon microphone was one such technology. It was initially developed for use in phones, but the design of the diaphragm was somewhat different in the hearing aids. The invention of the modern hearing aid may be said to have started with the telephone, and of course involving the famous, and partially deaf, inventor Thomas Edison, but the history of the telephone, the radio, surveillance and even taking pictures are interwoven.

Carbon hearing aids were available from about 1902, but they were heavy, clumsy and slow to catch on with hard of hearing people. As a result, acoustical hearing aids, like the speaking tube, remained popular. It was possible to get an ear trumpet through the British NHS into the 1970s, although by then there were alternatives. Still the carbon hearing aid was a milestone, and one on which the founding of at least one of the world's biggest hearing aid companies was originally based. If one man were to be singled out, it would be Miller Reese Hutchison, of New York, who founded The Akouphone Company in 1899, and who patented the first portable hearing aid in 1901. The hearing aid was small enough to be worn on a belt. His invention became famously significant, his hearing aid, which he called the Acousticon, was worn by the beautiful, but hearing impaired, Alexandra of Denmark, during her Coronation as the Queen of England in 1902.

The Acousticon comprised of three components, and the batteries lasted only a few hours. Presumably battery life was longer than the duration of the Coronation ceremony, and that the Royal Robes and Jewells were extensive enough to hide the contraption, but most importantly, Alexandra could hear enough. Interestingly, Hutchison, who was a great admirer of the work of Thomas Edison, and electro-acoustic engineering, is more famous for his invention of the Klaxon horn, which is a bit of an irony. Even the word Klaxon, which is from the Ancient Greek, *klázō* 'to shriek', or 'make a sharp sound'. He also went on to invent a conduction version called the Akoulallion. I rather like that name. Queen Alexandra, known to her family as Alix, was the daughter of Christian I of Denmark, and married Albert Edward Prince of Wales, when she was only 17. She started to lose her hearing not long after they were married, and she too suffered from otosclerosis, like my dad, and Beethoven, and Reynolds. Princess Alexandra was so pleased she awarded Hutchison a gold medal for Exceptional Merit in the Field of Innovation. Hutchison was invited to the Coronation, and the American press described his invention as 'a miracle' and 'the best electrical aid for the semi-deaf devised'. Hutchison partnered with Kelly Monroe Turner, who continued to develop and lead in hearing aid design, after Hutchison turned over the rights to the Acousticon and his company, The General Acoustic Company, to Turner in 1905. The

Acousticon was imported into Denmark about that time, and sold for about $60 US dollars, which equates to about $12,000.

Some companies maintain very high hearing aid prices today, and the reader is advised to do their homework on hearing aid prices. Products continued to improve, and to be associated with the name of Hutchinson, this moving passage was written about him by hard-of-hearing Lucy Taylor, it was published in *The Silent Worker* in 1913:

'It gave me the first ray of hope I have had in many years, for surely Mr. Hutchison knows what he is talking about. I have long felt, that if someone who understood, cared enough to really try, something might be invented, that would do for the partially deaf what glasses do for the partially blind – "hearing for the semi-deaf".'

There is yet another twist to the story of the hearing aid though, and this arises because of the legacy of Kelly Monroe Turner, one time president of the General Acoustics Company and inventor of the Dictaphone machine. Turner was predominantly interested in electro-acoustics, rather than hearing aids. He renamed his company Dictograph Products as his leading product became the great market success of the Dictograph. Kelly became most famous though, for the Detective Dictograph. This was vividly described in a 1912 edition of the *New York Daily Tribune* as: 'New Terror to Evildoers is that Scientific Eavesdropper, the Dictograph'. The intriguing subheading was:

'Use of Tiny Mechanical Detective Contrivance for the Recording of Supposed Secret Conversation, Between Suspected Parties in Famous Dynamiting and Bribery Cases Has Brought About a State of Mind Among Malefactor That Will Lead to a Careful Examination of All Furnishings and Attachments in Their Meeting Places'

The reporter visited Turner at his Long Island premises, and was fascinated by what he observed.

'It was an eerie experience to stand in a corner of Mr. Turner's office, far from a small wooden box, which was covered with a heavy overcoat, and whisper, "Do you hear me?" and receive a distinct, full bodied answer emanating from the box, the voice of someone in another part of the building, "Yes of course I hear you."'

Since the early work on electro-acoustic devices, research and development of audio surveillance and hearing aid devices have overlapped. However, the manufacturing and path to market have been very different. Apart from any ethical or philosophical views, which would direct researchers and manufacturers down very different paths, the cosmetic and technical requirements of a wearable aid to hearing, for an ear that doesn't process sound normally, are quite different to the requirements of a surveillance device. Despite this, I have been asked many times 'Could you use a hearing aid for spying?' And the answer is of course 'yes'. Meanwhile, a Danish entrepreneur, called William Demant became a major reseller of the Acousticon, laying the foundation for the Danish hearing aid industry.

The history of the first vacuum tube hearing aids overlaps with the carbon aid. Just as William Demant had been motivated to find a solution to his wife's increasing hearing loss, Edward Myers founded E.A.Myers & Sons, later called Radioear. Edward Myers was a criminal trial lawyer who lost much of his hearing and needed a solution for courtroom work. After years of collaboration, including a significant collaboration with a Western Electric engineer to find a suitable solution, a 185 lb, cabinet version of the first Radioear hearing aid, based on crystal radio technology was turned on in 1924. The hearing aid was responsive to a wider range of frequencies than the carbon tube hearing aid, and had better sound quality, but was not very portable.

The vacuum tube hearing aid was patented and commercially produced in the 1920s by American Earl. C. Hanson. Known as the Vacuphone, it was basically a carbon hearing aid using a Western Electric 205-A peanut tube (vacuum tube) for amplification. It was manufactured as a collaborative effort between the Western Electric Company and the Globe Phone Manufacturing Company. It used a telephone transmitter to convert sound into electrical signals. The downside of this new hearing aid was that it needed two big, expensive batteries, so there were challenges with this new development, which exemplified the development of hearing aids to the modern day – there is an ongoing requirement for better and yet smaller hearing aids.

The social environment was also changing in the 1920s. Interest in hearing loss and deafness had increased following the First World War. In Britain, the National Institute for the Deaf gained traction. Originally founded by Leo Bonn, a deaf merchant banker, and known as The National Bureau for Promoting the General Welfare of the Deaf in London, it became the National Institute for the Deaf in 1924. The Royal National Institute for Deaf People (RNID), more recently re-launched as Action on Hearing Loss, which is a charity working with Britain's 9 million people who are deaf or have hearing loss. Alongside its role in influencing public policy in favour of people who are hard of hearing in the UK, it also developed a role as a provider of care to deaf and hard of hearing people with additional needs during the late 1920s and early 1930s.

Military conflict generally speeds technology development. Hearing aids moved forward again before and just after the Second World War. Electronic circuitry and battery technology both took a step forward under the need for improved technology. These were both later utilised in the path towards more reliable and smaller hearing aids, where the batteries and electronics, including the microphone, were in a single unit. The earpiece was attached by a wire – a style that would remain unchanged for many years. The main body of the hearing aid was now small enough to fit into a man's top pocket in his jacket. Women would often clip the main body of the hearing aid to their underwear.

A further step forward came when the Bell Telephone Laboratories, released the transistor in 1948. This was another wartime development, as a version of the transistor had been patented much earlier, but interest was re-activated in radar research. Intense research and development efforts combined to lead to the transistor. The initial invention operated as a speech amplifier with a power gain of 18 in the first trial. In 1956, the co-inventors of the Transistor, John Bardeen, Walter Houser Brattain and William Shockley were honoured with the Nobel Prize in Physics 'for their researches on semiconductors and their discovery of the transistor', such was it's importance. There was a period where hobbyist electronics engineers were working with new products, where about 50 years later, they would be building small computers. Indeed, William Shockley's influence was one of the influences in the establishment of Silicon Valley, from which later the likes of Steve Jobs would emerge. Unfortunately relations between the three inventors deteriorated, but an American electrical engineer, by the name of Norman Krim, who worked at Raytheon, saw the potential of transistors to transform hearing aids, Raytheon's business model was to gain a licence from Bell Labs to sell transistors to hearing aid companies. The invention of the transistor reduced the power requirement to a level which enabled the aids incorporating their own batteries, to be reduced in size. The body of the aid, though somewhat smaller, was still worn, usually, on the chest, and was still connected to a separate earpiece.

The hearing aid industry suddenly took off. Technology was better and more wearable. A *Time Magazine* article in 1953 stated:

'This little device, a single speck of germanium, is smaller than a paper clip and works perfectly at one-tenth the power needed by the smallest vacuum tube. Today, much of Raytheon's transistor output goes to America's hearing aid industry.'

But there was more happening, in that there was a drive to post war compensation and welfare. In Britain, the National Health Service was formed, and the Royal National Institute for the Deaf, the RNID, successfully campaigned for the provision of free hearing aids. Initially, health secretary Aneurin Bevan opened the first NHS hospital in 1948, hospitals, doctors, nurses, pharmacists, opticians and dentists were brought together under one umbrella organisation, with salaried staff to provide services that would be free for all at the point of delivery, paid for by the tax payer. Thanks to the RNID, there were also to be specialist ear clinics at which patients could get an expert opinion and if needed a hearing aid. This set the path to auditory rehabilitation in Britain on a strongly medical model, which is not mirrored in all countries. It's quite different in Australia, where Government hearing aid provision, which is not universal, is through a non-medical agency.

In the USA, although universal healthcare is still a controversial concept, there was a move to rehabilitate the hearing of returning veterans. Audiology was established during the Second World War to treat veterans who came home and were suffering from hearing loss. Between 1945 and 1947, 15,000 veterans were seen for hearing loss, 45,000 by 1949 and 71,000 veterans were identified to have hearing loss by 1957. The Veterans Association began in the late 1950s.

Hearing aids changed remarkably little in the next 30 years. Eventually, improved miniaturisation techniques produced the behind-the-ear aid, many of them now discrete and elegant. Small, aids, are to be worn in the ear canal, so that they are invisible. These are now available, although the user has to be aware of the different trade-offs for sound quality, physical comfort and battery lifetime. Still, as early as the end of the 1950s, Otarion Electronics, in Chicago, introduced the first hearing aid worn entirely at the ear – the Otarion Listener. The company did this by putting the electronics in the temple pieces of a pair of eyeglasses. By 1959, 'hearing glasses' had captured about half the market. The glasses were even worn by people with perfect eyesight.

So now we know that all those trendy people wearing plain lens glasses for fashion, are actually using hearing aids, secretly. The trouble with combining glasses and hearing aids is that you can't hear when you have taken your glasses off.

The NHS designed and manufactured their own hearing aid. By December 1948, according to the Medical journal, *The Lancet*, 'more than 3000 of the hearing-aids designed by the electro-acoustics committee of the Medical Research Council have so far been distributed through the NHS'. Today, with competition in hearing aid manufacture, it seems incredible that the NHS effectively built their own hearing aids, known as 'Medresco' aids. This was a strategy followed by Australia as well. The original Medresco hearing aids were vacuum tube hearing aids. In December 1948 The Medresco aid was designed by the Medical Research Council before the NHS service was launched. It was developed by the Post Office Engineering Research Station at Dollis Hill, near London and assembled by a number of radio manufacturers. Although they knew that the market was large the Medresco aids, though cheap, were also already old fashioned, and did not use the latest technology. Transistors, incorporated into commercial hearing aids from 1953, were not used in the NHS until many years later.

From *The Lancet*:

'The microphone and valve circuit are housed in a small plastic container, while the batteries are in a separate leather pack – a little bulky because the batteries are designed to give a long service.'

This is what my father had to say about his Medresco hearing aid from the 1950s:

'I took delivery of my first hearing aid from Guy's Hospital and took it to my parent's home where I happened to be staying. It was a huge three-part affair – the main gizmo clipped on to my shirt front under my

tie, a great leather satchel of batteries hung from a belt or was stuffed into a trouser pocket, and there were coils of wire to sort out. So I sat down in the evening under a window overlooking the garden to try it out. Put it all together, got the ear mould into the ear and switched it on.'

This account has concentrated on what the hearing aid looked like, and not what they sounded like. This is what my dad, a young man in his 20s heard, when he turned it on:

'Nothing. Absolute silence. (The truth is that there wasn't any noise to listen to). Turned up the volume control a bit. Still nothing. Turned it up nearly full strength. And just then my father walked past outside the window pushing his old lawnmower with steel wheels along the concrete path. Wow! I thought the roof had fallen in.'

Dad's early Medresco hearing aid would have been a linear hearing aid, without any processing for noise management. Technology is very different today, although most people still need time to adjust to having artificial hearing. However, the fact that they were still bulky, and didn't sound good, put the hearing aid program into question. A 1952 survey carried out for the Ministry of Health and summarized in *The Lancet*, reported that the average daily use of the Medresco was 4.9 hours, and that only 18 per cent of the aids issued were ever taken to work. Health economists questioned whether this was an effective program, and whether the funds should be re-allocated. What an amazing piece of bureaucratic logic. The hearing aids don't work very well, so let's abandon the program. I fear that kind of logic continues today. Hearing aids are not all the same. There's a wide range of sound quality difference, depending on the technology used. Fortunately for my dad, he could afford a hearing aid from a private dispenser and he moved to a more contemporary model.

Australia had its own government hearing aid too. One of the great pioneers of Australian technology and research into hearing was Dr Laurie Upfold. He was an Australian with a big influence on hearing aid, he ascribed the need for the development of Government hearing aid services in Australia, not just to the war, and returning servicemen, but also to the Australia wide rubella epidemic of the early 1940s. Maternal German measles (rubella), in the first or second trimester frequently causes severe hearing loss, as hearing develops very early in the gestational period. The need for two quite different types of service led to the development of the Commonwealth Acoustic Laboratories (CAL). In June 1948, the Laboratories were given Royal ascent '... for scientific investigation including that in respect of hearing aids and their application to the needs of individuals, and in respect of problems with noise as it affects individuals.'

Service provision came through Australian Hearing, and the research arm eventually became the National Acoustic Laboratories. The first CAL aid was similar to the first Medresco aid. It was designed and manufactured by the Commonwealth Acoustic Laboratories. It was a body worn style, with a button earphone attached by a cord. The aid was based on three valves, and used a piezoelectric microphone and electro magnetic earphone. It had three tone controls to emphasise either the high or the low frequencies. The Australians were quicker to move to a transistor hearing aid than the British, and introduced the CAL aid T in 1955. This new CAL aid was still a body worn hearing aid, but it was smaller, more reliable and more robust, batteries also lasted longer than previous CAL aid models. The hearing aid satisfied much current thinking about hearing aids, and left much legacy thinking that is no longer true, such as a view that a hearing aid frequency cut off at 4 kHz is satisfactory, it isn't. The view was probably influenced by the requirements for telephone handsets. This, and other hearing aids of the time, were really only suitable for people who had quite severe hearing loss, which affected most frequencies similarly.

One of the troubles with a body-worn hearing aid is the position of the microphone, which was generally built into the top, or the top front, of the hearing aid. That's not where your ears are, so it's very different to a normal listening experience. When I worked at the Royal National Throat, Nose and Ear Hospital, lots of patients, even in the early 1980s were still using body worn hearing aids, the microphones endured environments that had little in common with an ear level microphone.

The goal then was to get hearing aids to be small and light enough that they could be worn at ear level. The race was on. But, it wasn't as easy as it might sound because designers were simultaneously trying to improve the hearing aid sound quality and efficacy. There is of course debate as to the first manufacturer to produce a 'Behind the Ear' hearing aid. BTE hearing aids, began appearing around 1956 although probably the first BTE hearing aid made – Sonotone's Model 79 – came out in June of 1955. Dahlberg came out with their Model D-12 in February 1956. The 'Diplomat' was hearing aid manufacturer Zenith Radio, of Chicago's first BTE hearing aid. It came onto the market in June 1956. The 'Diplomat' used four transistors and had an external button speaker. The case measured 2¾" by ¾" and was sometimes referred to as the 'Banana' because of its large size. In 1964, Zenith sold a behind-the-ear model using an integrated circuit amplifier and a 1.2-volt button battery. It weighed just 7 grams, and Zenith claimed it was 500 times more reliable than hearing aids built with discrete transistors. In Australia, the Commonwealth Acoustic Laboratory skipped this stage and went directly to a hearing aid built completely into a moulded earpiece (an in the ear hearing aid).

The challenge my dad described when he was surprised by the lawnmower was a result of the linearity of those early hearing aids, coupled with some of the effects of hearing loss. When hearing deteriorates the ability to hear, soft sounds deteriorate, but loud sounds stay about the same loudness. Imagine a picture, the 'soft' parts of the picture are lost, the loud parts are not. The ear codes loudness faster than normal. Early hearing aids just made sounds louder. The challenge for the manufacturer was to stop them getting too loud without distorting the sound. When I was a student at Manchester University in the mid 1970s I learnt that you had to somehow 'chop off' the sound if it got too loud. The choices were simply 'how?' How to limit the output of the hearing aids without increasing distortion. Even in the 1970s, hearing aid scientist and inventor, Mead Killion, wrote that hearing aid distortion was sometimes so bad that people with normal hearing had problems when they tried to listen to speech in background noise.

Linear hearing aids are called 'linear' because they amplify all sounds by the same amount. It seems obvious that what was needed was a non-linear hearing aid – one that wouldn't keep getting louder as sounds got louder. But how loud should they be anyway? The answer surely should be 'loud enough, but comfortable'. After many years of research, hearing scientists are still not in agreement on the best hearing aid output parameters, or how to achieve them. By the 1940s, testing the sensitivity of hearing by measuring the softest sound you can hear at a range of frequencies, in a padded room or tiny phone box-like capsule, had become popular, if not standard. This became known as the pure tone audiogram.

It was not at all obvious for many years how to set up hearing aids so that they would be audible and comfortable. This isn't surprising. The pure tone audiogram measures the softest sounds you can hear in a background of near silence. Hearing aids need to process and transmit the right sound to you, in a diverse range of backgrounds that are constantly changing. With some hearing aids, that's still a challenge today. Since the early days of audiology, in the 1940s, the science of how to set up, or personalise a hearing aid has progressed hand in hand with changes in hearing aid technology. There was actually an interesting technique developed in the 1930s, although its origins are earlier, using a Master Hearing Aid.

The first 'fitting methods', as personalisation of hearing aids became known, were devised for linear hearing aids – hearing aids that amplified all sounds by the same amount at any one frequency. An internal limit is imposed that restricts the transmission of very loud sounds, by clipping the peak of the sound. That causes distortion, which markedly reduces the quality of listening.

In 1946, Raymond Carhart developed a way of setting up hearing aids using speech sounds, but clinicians thought that this left too much to individual judgement and they sought a numerical prescription that took them from the beep test (pure tone audiogram) to the hearing aid setting. Given that hearing aids generally came pre-set up to the late 1970s, this was quite important as the clinician had to order the hearing aids with the amplification settings.

At first it seemed logical that the audiogram could be 'mirrored'. That is, we could put in as much amplification as there is hearing loss. Unfortunately this doesn't work because loudness perception grows abnormally quickly for people with inner ear hearing loss. People with sensory neural hearing loss have a reduced dynamic range of hearing. The dynamic range, which is different across the range of perceptible frequencies, is the difference in dB between the softest sound someone can hear and the sound that they find on the uncomfortable side of loud. The dynamic range can be quite small for some pitch sounds and quite large for others. It depends on the pattern of damage in the cochlea. It's as if the floor and the ceiling have got closer together, but to different degrees.

From the 1940s over the next forty years, scientists proposed a number of different rules, but they all suffered from two main problems: the first is that there is a fundamental problem in having hearing aids with amplification that's the same for the whole range of input sounds. The second problem is that it relies on people liking the outcome of formula for listening levels that's based on averages. Imagine being given an average shoe size, if you don't happen to be the average. Most hearing aids today are non-linear.

Because hearing impaired people usually have the abnormally rapid and nonlinear loudness growth that I've described, then most modern hearing aids have a compressive amplifier. The theory of this is that it restores the nonlinearity by amplifying soft sounds more than loud sounds. This would remain the case till we later solved the problem.

To automatically control the gain electronically, the incoming sound level is detected and amplified by different amounts, depending on the intensity of the incoming sound. The theory is that a normal cochlear would amplify soft sounds more than loud sounds, and that the hearing aid should do the same. Not all scientists are in agreement on this theory. My theory is that everyone is different.

In 1948, Multitone of London produced the first hearing aid with automatic gain control (AGC), but it was a tabletop model, as the increased power requirement had not been solved.

A major development in the history of hearing aids was the zinc-air battery. This battery is mercury free and has a greater capacity than the mercury battery because of the greater volume of the anode. The smaller zinc-air batteries propel development and sales of ITE (in-the-ear) hearing aids. I finished my master's degree in audiology that year. I had no idea that such a revolutionary discovery had been made. Sometimes, the narrow world of the universities miss the big picture. This was one of those times.

The story of the development of non-linear hearing aids, moves on to Wide Dynamic Gain Compression (WDRC), a particular kind of AGC, and with the interaction of developments in telephony continuing, hearing aid researchers had observed the successful use of WDRC transatlantic phone cables, as early as the 1930s.

The Medical Acoustic Instrument Company Inc of Minneapolis, which became known as Maico is now a major manufacturer of audiology equipment, and they manufactured and released the Maico hearing aid Model AO in 1960. This was a 6-transistor hearing aid with AGC (automatic gain control). It was made of stainless steel over black plastic and was relatively compact, measuring 6.6cm x 4.45cm x 0.6cm thick – smaller than an iPhone, though thicker. The Maico Model AO used two 1.4-volt mercury batteries. A cord attached to the hearing aid speaker, which was clipped to a customised earpiece. The trend to reduced size continued and the first high quality behind the ear (BTE) hearing aid was sold in about 1965.

At this stage, clinicians were not sure how to properly personalise these non-linear hearing aids for each individual. The starting information was the softest sound that the user could hear and the level of sound that they find uncomfortable sounds. This slowed the adoption of non-linear hearing aids. I studied audiology in 1975 and non-linear hearing aids barely got a mention on my master's degree course. I did learn that compression limiting was an alternative to peak clipping as a means of avoiding excessive output. But by the early 1970s scientists were demonstrating the benefits of WDRC, compared with linear hearing aids. The research showed that people were hearing better in background noise, and found loud sounds less disturbing. The next challenge then for the non-linear hearing aid was to find a consumer friendly implementation.

The precise path of the incorporation and widespread transition to non-linear hearing aids is interwoven with changes in circuitry, the introduction of partial digital solutions, changes in style of hearing aids, and miniaturisation. The progress is characterised by commercial product releases, technology comparisons, as researchers gathered evidence and formed opinions about the types of technologies and the best way to use them; education of audiologists and the influence of government distribution contracts and procedures. These factors still influence, and to some extent hold back, new developments today. The timing of new developments is such that there are hearing aid users who equate the move to digital, with the move to compression, and who are convinced that the old analogue hearing aids are better than any digital aid could be. I am not the only audiologist who has lost sleep over this problem, puzzling how to convince these clients of the need to change. I read this on a UK blog recently and have quoted it verbatim, below:

'A few years ago the audiology dept in Liverpool tried to issue me with the new generation of analogue/digital devices, and I couldn't use them as they cut out the sounds I wish to hear, as they have new devices within them called active gain control and a compressor. Natural hearing works on an analogue level. There is no such thing as a digital sound, the only thing digital in hearing aids is the processor, aid converter, and d/a converter. The input and output stages are still analogue.'

I have never met this person, but feel as though I have, as I meet this issue often, but I can't agree with everything he says. The issues pointed out in the first paragraph have nothing to do with digital technology – active gain control and compression were first implemented in analogue devices.

Let's have a quick recap of what's actually going on here: in an analogue hearing aid, the microphone picks up the sound and converts it into an electrical input signal. This signal is amplified and some spectral shaping is done. The amplified signal is converted by the loudspeaker ('receiver' in hearing-aid-speak) back to an acoustic signal. The acoustic and the electrical signals can be thought of as being continuous in time. This is like thinking of the continuous sound profile stored along a groove on a vinyl record.

An analogue hearing aid is full of capacitors and transistors; a digital hearing aid has a very small, but quite powerful, computer in it to process the signals. This provides a lot of opportunity to 'do things better'.

In the digital hearing aid, the microphone still converts the acoustic signal to an electrical signal, but then an analogue-to-digital converter converts the electrical signal into a series of numbers that represent the amplitude of the signal. The number of times that this happens affects the fidelity of the digitised signal. This is referred to as sampling. The small computer can then carry out sophisticated signal processing, and hearing aid engineers work to make sure that sophisticated processes can be performed without too much power drain on the battery.

The transition from analogue to digital, in hearing instruments, was gradual, and started with digital control over the hearing aid controls, so that the hearing aid could be described as 'programmable'. In the next stage of development, much of the hearing aid circuitry was replaced by a tiny computer chip.

There have been some standout developments in the path to widespread adoption of non-linear hearing aids, and in particular compression in the late 1980s. During this period, the first multi-channel hearing aids appeared, and the earliest digital hearing aids were released. The path to a feasible, small hearing aid was getting easier, and the nearly invisible, 'In The Canal' (ITC) hearing aids were introduced in 1989. According to the Hearing Industries Association (HIA) statistical report, digital signal processing (DSP) hearing aids became the most common hearing aid sold in the U.S.A. during the first quarter of 2002, passing both digitally programmable analogue and non-programmable hearing aids.

CHAPTER FOURTEEN

HEARING DYNAMICALLY – THE NEXT BIG THING IN HEARING AIDS

Where else would you go, in Australia, to reignite a career in hearing research, but the Bionic Ear Institute? The Bionic Ear Institute was a wonderful place to work, but perhaps the best thing was that I didn't know that there were always more helpful and exciting developments in store for people with hearing loss. After the success with the new electrode it was time for a new project. A leading researcher in both cochlear implant technology and children's hearing and language, invented a new way to amplify sound in hearing aids, that would control the loudness better than in other hearing aid, and wouldn't distort sound so much. In other words, he had seen how to solve the problems that compression introduced to hearing aids, and had found a better way to control loudness, without the distortion. It later turned out that this combination also helped people hear better in background noise. His name is Peter Blamey, and he has been my research colleague and business partner for 15 years now.

Professor Peter Blamey had been working on a research project to help people who wanted to use both a cochlear implant in one ear and a hearing aid in the other ear to hear as well as possible. His team also wanted to find a way of setting up the combined hearing aid and cochlear implant duo, very easily and by the same professional. Can you believe that in some parts of the world, even today, if you have a hearing aid in one ear and a cochlear implant in the other, then your ears effectively belong to different clinicians, possibly in different establishments? This needn't be the case. Although the method of getting sound to the hearing nerves is quite different, it turns out that the most important thing is to get the sensation of loudness to be the same in each ear. Cochlear implants are designed to be set up to comfortable loudness, hearing aids should be too, but have been evolved down this slightly strange path of predicting what sound level a certain hearing loss should be – on average, that is, whilst using various types of compression amplifiers to achieve non linearity. It was clearly going to be difficult to have a measure of loudness comfort in one ear and a prediction of sound output based on a hearing threshold in the other with that system. Peter was also puzzled that hearing scientists were prolific in discussing the problems of using compression in hearing aids and yet continued to do so. It so happened that Peter Blamey invented something new, and I became involved in a new chapter of helping people hear better.

Peter and his team knew they had invented the next important step in hearing aid technology. They had invented the next amplifier. Compression hearing aids were about to be part of the history of hearing aids. Life can seem very simple when there is a big discovery or invention and you don't have to worry about the power of advertising and commerce. Of course life isn't that simple. This was not going to get into lots of hearing aids by being written about in an academic journal. So we decided to start a company. For years the cochlear implant researchers at the Bionic Ear Institute had been using digital signal processing strategies to create hearing through the cochlear implant. Computer technology had moved on. A little company in Canada, the DSP Factory, was designing digital processors, in the same family as those used in cochlear implants, but which were very small and would run with very small batteries.

The DSP Factory designed ultra-low power DSP chips intended for use in hearing aids. Hearing aid companies today are really chip designers, and the intention at the DSP Factory had been to fulfil that role in the industry. We thought that if there was a company designing computer chips for hearing aids and we were writing clever software for hearing aids that there were obvious parallels and this would be a match made in heaven. Things didn't work out quite that way, but I really admire the work of Rob Brennan, Todd Schneider and their colleagues in Canada, who were really the ones responsible for a new era in hearing aids.

DSP Factory Ltd was a start up in Canada in the late 1990s. Their early product, the Toccata DSP chip was a technology that changed the hearing aid industry forever, because researchers from around the world could implement the latest research in hearing aids onto this powerful and tiny computer. The hearing aid world was no longer the preserve of a handful of giant multi-national hearing aid companies.

We now had the opportunity to use our digital signal processing in hearing aids. To understand the impact, let's go back to the cochlear implant for a minute. A cochlear implant processor takes real world sound and converts it to a digitised signal. Then the digitised signal is mathematically manipulated to make the signal more useful to the user. As time has gone on the mathematical manipulation has become more and more sophisticated, to improve the hearing and listening experience. The miniature processor carries out all the mathematical calculations, very quickly. Some mathematical processes take a lot more battery power than others. We've seen how important discrete hearing aids are to the user, so for hearing aids we needed to invent clever calculations that makes the world sound good, but didn't need a big battery. We didn't need to do things the old way anymore. We could invent hearing aid processing that didn't have the problems of compression.

I've written about the loudness challenge for hearing aid users and hearing aid developers. People with hearing loss have a reduced range of loudness perception, which has traditionally been addressed by analogue compression circuits. We needed to use these tiny computers and clever mathematics to solve other problems too. Remember when hearing aids used to squeal a lot? One of the most important inventions for hearing aids has been the introduction of excellent feedback cancellation technology. This is one of the areas where the mathematical manipulation could use a lot of power, so all the main manufacturers do things a little bit differently to try to get rid of most of the squealing, without having to have a bigger battery, and hence a bigger hearing aid. But I'm getting ahead of myself.

We decided to start a company. Naivety can be a wonderful thing it makes it much harder to spot obstacles. We entered the Melbourne Business School Entrepreneurs Challenge, a business competition, and won it, and in the process attracted venture capital. I don't think anyone in the hearing aid industry expected us to last six months. Fourteen years later, the company is going strong, and its 'graduates' are working around the globe.

I'll skip about a years' worth of wrangling with the University, which was painful, and jump to the point where Peter and I found ourselves leading a company, essentially owned by Venture Capital and developing sound processing software for hearing aids. Our Life Sciences investors proposed that we go out to the hearing aid companies and licence the new amplifier. They were strongly of the view that we needed a high royalty rate for the use of the amplifier in hearing aids. It is not uncommon in biotech business for any licensee to buy the licensor, thus avoiding the need to pay future royalties and acquiring a valuable asset. It became clear early on this was not going to work in the hearing aid business. The appetite for large royalties was non-existent. The vision to sell this amazing new amplifier, which by then had been named Adaptive Dynamic Range Optimisation or ADRO® for short, and other technologies too, to customers of the DSP Factory, that is people using the DSP processing chips was underway. The only point in developing hearing aid sound processing is to sell it to hearing aid companies. Rather oddly, I had been so engrossed in the goal, that I had somehow not thought very hard about the fact that all the hearing aid companies were overseas, and a long way from Australia.

By this time I had eased into the role of being in charge of a very innovative start up company, with an overseas customer base and I also had four children aged from nine to fourteen. It wasn't long after this that my husband John took charge of running the family, which wasn't a very easy step at the beginning of the noughties, because there were so few men in that role. No sitcoms on househusbands then. He did a great job, but I found it hard to spend so much time at work, or away, or to hear my child say, 'Well, you're hardly ever here, but when you are, you're thinking about work.' Once I came home a bit early in the day, and my daughters were so surprised to find me in the kitchen cooking dinner, that they asked me if I'd been fired. Then the eldest, wisely, but sadly said. 'You're having a guilt attack: actually we can manage. Please get out of the kitchen.'

Meanwhile, whilst overseeing clinical trials of the new amplifier, and building a team of audiologists and engineers, it was time to meet the customers. Peter and I went visiting hearing aid companies. We started, logically, at the DSP Factory.

The DSP Factory was a couple of years older than us, so I was excited to learn of their experiences in changing the world. They were great people, and very kind to us. We were all filled with optimism, though we also laid some groundwork in how the financial split would be divided between software (us) and hardware (them), the assumption being, wrongly as it turned out, that any hearing aid company would be prepared to spend a certain amount on the combination. Investors, who wanted to see a timely return on their investment, funded both Dynamic Hearing and the DSP Factory. We were about to come face to face, with the phrase 'Make versus Buy', which is much more than a straightforward cost of goods decision.

The DSP Factory was in Waterloo, in Canada, which is in a beautiful area in summer and very cold, for Australians, in winter. We visited and were looked after well, worked out our business model; discovered the enchanting Niagara by the Lake, and found out what it was like to enjoy the business partnership of thoroughly nice people. The DSP Factory got acquired, and its acquirer got acquired, but we collectively changed an industry, raised the standards of hearing aids, and made some good friends. There are hotspots of activity in hearing aid research, development and manufacture, Ontario is one of them. Of course, it's not all coincidence – it's more a case of staff leaving one entity to start another. But I am happy that this particular hotspot showed us St. Jacob's, with its colourful market and influence of the Mennonite people, the Niagara region, and its lovely produce. Between the DSP Factory and us, we kept pushing technology forward.

Our next obvious step was to find the customers of the DSP Factory. I decided the most likely customer for us was a company called Intrason, in Paris. Not only did they use the DSP Factory chip, they had been the first to use it. I knew lots about hearing aid signal processing and cochlear implant development; I was a good audiologist; I knew we had the world's best technology, but I was in Melbourne, in a start-up environment with only a few staff, and had never built a hearing aid. Hmm: Where to start? 'Well', I thought, 'The obvious thing to do is to have a French lesson.' So I did. I felt much better after that, and armed with a few years of schoolgirl French, and the intensive refresher, I rang Intrason, in Paris. I was lucky that my schoolgirl French only had to get me through the switchboard, which had been a major object of the French lesson. I explained my proposal. What's much more exciting – they liked my proposal. The French do have a reputation for innovation. 'But you are in Australia. How will this work?' It was a Monday. 'I can be there on Friday to explain.' I said, with no idea at all of whether I could get a flight to get me to Paris by Friday. I did, and by Wednesday night, Peter and I were on our way to Paris, and we came back with a commission to provide the entire signal processing for a new hearing aid.

Our little team was fantastic. The Intrason engineers were great to work with, they were enthusiastic and they embraced our new technologies. However, it also seemed that they were under some financial stress, having expanded very rapidly. Our remit was to help them get out the next product extremely quickly. We did it: our team rose to the occasion in a magnificent way. It was wonderful to witness the excitement of the research and engineering team in Australia, seeing their inventions go to help people with hearing problems, rather than lying in a dusty journal. As we might have expected the hearing aid was received well, the new amplifier had been proven in clinical trials, so we could write about it in marketing material. It was a success, and actor Jean Lefebvre publicly endorsed the hearing aid. Unfortunately, Intrason was not such a success. The hearing aid sold well, but we were too late. They had overstretched their resources so many of the staff went on to work in other hearing aid companies in France and we found ourselves with friends and contacts who would help us on our way to more relationships.

The hearing aid companies are generally in nice places, while mostly quite a long way apart. We visited them all, and got to know the heads of technology in each of them. We felt it was important to make our customers feel that we were near at hand. We in Australia know that we have to travel to do business, and I came to think of Los Angeles or Singapore as the next stops as one might think of the next train stop as your nearest town.

I think people in Europe and in America tend to think that we are a long way away. I wanted to minimise this feeling. So we travelled to Denmark and Switzerland and the United States many, many times. An American colleague once referred to us as the hardest working people in the hearing aid industry. My favourite place to do business was Japan. It is such a beautiful and interesting country and I greatly respect the Japanese people that I worked with, and their style of doing business.

We realised quite quickly that we had to design more than just an amplifier. It would be easier to sell signal processing for a whole hearing aid system. So we designed an operating framework, much like the one you have in your computer, to run on the tiny DSP Factory's chip. Then we designed solutions that would also fit in the operating system (OS), to solve other hearing aid technical problems, such as the need for hearing aids to minimise whistling. It's a bit like designing different software packages to fit in with the Microsoft or Apple operating systems. We could work with a company to provide a 'pick and mix' feature improvement. This made our business very flexible. We raised more money from our venture capitalists to do this, and we were also fortunate in being awarded some government grants. I'm happy to say that we more than repaid these in export revenue. The team was then able to design operating systems for other chips. This meant that once the OS was in place on another chip we could implement technologies quite easily, this gave us the opportunity to go into other business areas than hearing aids. It was now possible to supply technology to headset phone companies and we managed to build a very strong relationship with a company in the United States. As time went on more and more headset manufacturing moved to Southeast Asia. I rather liked this as Australia is nearer to Southeast Asia than Europe.

A modern hearing aid is a mixture of good mechanical design and smart signal processing on the computer chip. Now that we had a whole hearing aid system running in software on a DSP computer chip, we could access that chip in other hearing aids and turn it effectively into a new hearing aid quite quickly. At this point hearing aid designers were taking about six months to develop a new hearing aid. We demonstrated to German company Interton, a hearing aid company based near Cologne, that if they worked with us a new hearing aid could be developed in about an hour. We told them that we could convert their hearing aid into a completely new hearing aid quite quickly. I don't think they were convinced, they used the DSP Factory chip in their hearing aids so Peter took one of their hearing aids back to our hotel after our day visit and between 5 o'clock and 6 o'clock he converted it into a brand-new hearing aid with our technologies. He even had time for a nap. When our hosts picked us up for dinner that evening we presented them with a brandnew hearing aid, they were impressed. This was the beginning of a partnership that lasted for several years. Again, we made good friends and built a solid collaboration. We recognised that making an excellent hearing aid needs both excellent signal processing and excellent mechanical design. Interton had excellent mechanical design.

Interton was a medium-size hearing company, which became a very fast growing company, partly as a result of our collaboration. This, however, sealed their fate as an acquisition target and now this wonderful technology team has been partly absorbed and partly disbanded as a result of being acquired by a larger company.

One of my favourite stories took place when we received a call from a hearing company in Salt Lake City, at the time we were staying in Silicon

Valley. It seemed like an important call so we got on a plane the next day. It was a fine day when we left San Francisco and we were so pleased to be travelling without full suitcases that we didn't even think to take a coat. When we landed in Salt Lake City the snow was driving hard, it was a whiteout! After an extraordinary, taxi ride in which we gained more sound memories, with colourful African music playing, while the snow fell heavily outside, we finally arrived at our meeting, needless to say we were extremely late, be it with a good story to tell. The visit was successful, and we had helped another hearing aid company.

During these years, I learned a lot about what people need from their hearing aids and what people need from headsets. I learnt that hearing aid companies appear to adopt new technologies and that headset companies, that will focus on their customers, adopt new technologies very quickly. It seemed to me that hearing aid companies saw the audiologist as their customer, rather than the hearing aid user. In writing the tales of technology sales though, what comes to mind are the stories of places and the people we met. Although we spent many weekends away, I was always reluctant to not work. Somehow it seemed wrong to be away from my family and not working, I was new to business, so I wanted to make sure that I really did my best. I wanted to make Dynamic Hearing successful, and I wasn't good at taking weekends off when travelling, or at home. A typical weekend afternoon during a business trip might be to find a nice cafe to go work in.

We worked closely with some Japanese companies, both on hearing aids and on headsets. Our Japanese customers wanted to know every last detail of the path forward and the technology before they would consider making a commercial agreement. It made them a pleasure to work with because, by the time they had the picture to their satisfaction, we had built up good friendships and because they had developed such a strong understanding of both the business and the technology. Our Japanese colleagues were also enormously hospitable to us. In learning to be more informed about appropriate behaviour in Japanese business culture, we worked with a consultant, who was wonderful in advising me. On my first trip, we flew in from Canada. Tired and considerably jet lagged, I initially found the bustle of Tokyo a bit overwhelming, but I later found out what an amazing and diverse city it is. The first hotel we stayed at was enormous and seemed so impersonal, which led me to wonder if anyone would even know if I died of jet lag overnight – would I be found in the morning?

On one memorable occasion, I joined a trade mission to Osaka, which was organised by the Kansai chamber of Commerce. They arranged for me to visit an electronic component company in the west of Japan, who were interested in our headset technologies. This particular company is a major international supplier in that area to mobile phone manufacturers. I travelled with a business guide and an interpreter to a very imposing factory set in a rural area, some two hours train journey from Osaka. It was the most traditional company that I'd ever visited, even though it was a modern electronics components company. When we arrived, I had to swap my shoes for slippers. This didn't make me feel very business-like. We were ushered into a meeting room along with some engineers, and I prepared to show a presentation. The furniture arrangement in the meeting room was a little unusual in my experience of business meetings. The three of us were seated in a deep and comfortable settee opposite the engineers from the host company. The settees were decorated with white antimacassars. It's really not easy to feel corporate and confident, wearing slippers, sitting settled deeply into a settee, unless you are accustomed to that as a business setting. Tea was served in beautiful china teacups. I did my best with the presentation and with answering questions with the help of the interpreter. But things got worse. When we were waiting outside the factory for our taxi, I asked our interpreter for her impressions of the meeting. She told me that she thought the third engineer was really, really nice. At that point I wondered what their discussion had actually been about, and whether it had anything to do with consumer electronics. We didn't win an opportunity to do further business with that company, so I may never know.

We were very happy to see hearing aids with our technology on the market in Japan and to have continued opportunity to work there. We didn't just work with corporations in Japan. We also developed some research collaborations. We spent some time with academic researchers at the University in Osaka. On one occasion we were treated to a splendid dinner in the University Club. Outside, a typhoon was raging. The sky looked black, and the trees were horizontal. We were concerned that our guests may have needed to go home to support their families in such dangerous conditions. However, out of politeness the professor had asked all of his team to stay to dinner with us, and I formed the view that no one would have dreamt of going home early lest that be seen as poor behaviour.

Peter and I know that we have brought something quite new to the hearing aid industry. We have developed an operating system much like the Windows operating system that almost everyone is familiar with. We have developed modules of hearing aid signal processing that could be mixed and matched to make new hearing aids and Bluetooth headsets. We have shown that a small team of Australian engineers could make a big change in the quality of hearing aids. Most of the big hearing aid companies and headset companies around the world have tested our technologies and found them to be very good. Some purchased our technologies and collaborated with us for new products. Some of the very big hearing aid companies decided to make their own DSP chips, making the idea of the hearing aid world being dominated by an independent chip provider and an independent signal processing (software) provider, less possible. We had a good team and we were fast, this was definitely an important commercial asset. I got to know a lot of the senior business people in the hearing aid industry. My MBA got completed by learning on the job, negotiating with CEOs of multinationals. I mused that there might be room to develop a practical MBA course component: my students would be made to stay awake for 24 hours to simulate their airline experience and then do a sales presentation. I felt that it was important that our customers saw that it would be as easy to do business with us from Australia as it would be to do business with someone on the next street, distance was no barrier to collaboration. So I tried never to talk about things like time differences or season differences and to always look fresh and alert. I'm not sure, but I suspect that I generally succeeded.

I was surprised by the extent to which CEOs of major corporations would share commercial stories with me, especially when they had achieved a commercial success. This is how I learnt that it was more likely to be a cosmetic development rather than a better hearing development that brought the most commercial success in the hearing aid field, in their eyes.

I became a businesswoman, and in 2004 won the prestigious Telstra Businesswoman of the year competition, for the Corporate and Government sector. I would not have predicted this step a few years before. I came to understand the economic and business structure of the hearing aid industry and I formed strong views that much of it was not in the best interests of the consumer. The current structure leads to many people paying a great deal of money for their hearing aids, and to some components of the commercial chain getting a lot of profit at their expense. I have always wanted to make a difference to the lives of people with hearing loss. For me, that made making hearing aids better and more financially accessible. I was sure we could do better than the existing solutions, but to do that we had to be more in control of the whole product. I was also very interested in people being able to set up the parameters of their own hearing aids, and being more in control of their aids. I wanted to see the latest technologies going into hearing aids, more quickly. The hearing aid industry seemed to move so much more slowly than the headset industry. Indeed, the hearing aid industry was in danger of falling behind technologically. It became clear to me that Dynamic Hearing would be sold to a company in the telephony industry, not the hearing aid industry, because the telephony industry was moving faster, and needed a supply of good signal processing solutions. The hearing aid industry was shutting down to third party solutions like us. We had built an 'A' team of sound processing developers. I did my best to help sell the company, but to do this, I had mentally moved on. I didn't want to work for a phone company. So, I decided to move on to pursue my main interest of helping people with hearing problems.

Although I moved on to other things, I am really proud of what we achieved at Dynamic Hearing. Peter and I developed a reputation for hard work, persistence and problem solving in the hearing aid and headset industry. We spent a lot of time on planes and in Denmark, France, Switzerland, Japan, and the United States and in Southeast Asia. The experience of learning about consumer products as well as hearing aids was a vital experience that we brought into our later work. Our audiologists at Dynamic Hearing mostly moved on to senior business and audiology roles in the hearing aid industry when Peter and I moved on. Most of the major hearing aid companies tested our technologies and compared them to their own and none of them published the results. There is something to be deduced from that.

The DSP Factory made it possible for teams like ours to produce world leading hearing aid technology. The pace of development of signal processing in hearing aids accelerated very rapidly. Peter had for many years been developing and evaluating DSP solutions for cochlear implants – the impossible had now been made possible in hearing aids. For the person with hearing loss, this meant a lot of change, it meant there was no need for hearing aids to cost so much. The price of top quality hearing aids could come well down at the same time as the sound quality went up. Peter Blamey abandoned the traditional 30-year-old compression solution to amplifying sound via the hearing aid in order to make sound through hearing aids more natural.

I am quite confident that as a result of our work not only did new technologies get into the hearing aids of the world; we also pushed the bar higher. Large companies saw what a small, innovative team of scientists and engineers in Australia could do. In response, all hearing aid technology improved. Peter and I didn't make any financial return from Dynamic Hearing, other than our salaries, but we did leave a legacy we are proud of, including training and enhancing the career of several engineers and audiologists. Peter and I have maintained a commitment to helping young people develop skills and expertise, to encouraging students and contributing to the innovation ecosphere in Australia. My wonderful husband and children were supportive of my many overseas absences, and I think I can count myself an expert world traveller.

CHAPTER FIFTEEN

My own hearing aid company, and much more, at last

I try hard to understand the multitude of challenges faced by most people with hearing loss. Of course, they are all so different, depending on how much loss, when that loss occurred and a person's overall life style and circumstances. No two people have the same story. There is a big challenge for people who fall between the worlds of signing, oral, partial hearing, regular school, lifestyles, career hopes, and family relationships. However hard I try, I am sure that I won't ever fully understand. I do lots of advocacy to help raise awareness and I am involved in lots of volunteer projects. One day a young traveller to Australia, from England, contacted me to see who or what I knew about services for young people in Australia. As a person who is quite deaf, she has reached out to help other people form strategies to help manage their hearing loss, and their emotional life. Now I want to let Zoe tell her story:

ZOE'S STORY

'It is quite a shock when anyone realises that something about themselves is different. It is difficult too when you start to feel abnormal and decide to do nothing about it, or you do something

to try to fix it and still don't feel fixed. At the age of 14 I was diagnosed with a hearing loss worthy of hearing aids. I can't remember now what type of loss or how severe, however, it was implied that I would be able to get by without them so as a teenager I opted to avoid anything that was going to make me different from my friends. The ENT surgeon showed me that he himself also wore hearing aids but that they were very discreet because he was vain. As far as I was concerned they weren't discreet enough.

'It seems in fact that I was born with a hearing loss, though because my early hearing results were mislaid somewhere between my primary school and the hospital we are unsure what scale of hearing loss I had at a young age. The signs went unnoticed at home and at school. I was a sociable little girl and from the age of two apparently enjoyed long conversations with my parent's friends over the telephone, my vocabulary and speech seemed normal so although many have commented that they are surprised my parents didn't notice sooner, they really had very little to go on.

'However, when my behaviour started to change around the age of seven or eight they did notice. I was more erratic and frustrated and became very anxious, particularly at school. My mother even took time off work to help in my class as an assistant to see if that would help her understand the problem. Finally, because it seemed that I was struggling most while I was at school, it was decided that I would go and see a specialist who might be able to diagnose me more successfully. We were told that I had "mild dyslexic tendencies" which just meant that they didn't know what was wrong with me either, however they did suggest that a school with smaller classes might help.

'At the age of nine I was moved to a new school and there did seem to be some improvement though something still wasn't quite right. As the television slowly grew louder and my imagination became increasingly colourful as I misheard more and more it started to become clearer. My parents decided to find out if I had ever failed a hearing test before. It turned out that I had but that they had never been told. By this point I was at my third and final school.

'The upshot of the conversation we had with the ENT surgeon was that I was pretty deaf but should probably be able to carry on unaided since I'd done alright so far. This was a rather mixed blessing because although I interpreted this as him telling me I was disabled, at least it was an "invisible" disability that I would be able to hide from my friends.

'There were certain moments of embarrassment throughout school that resulted as a consequence of my hearing. There are few that I can remember now but some still feel quite vivid. One day after swimming my classmates and I were all getting dressed. One girl said something and then disappeared, I followed her because I hadn't heard what she said and was greeted by her being almost completely naked. It turned out that she had instructed no one to come round the corner. We were both bright red and embarrassed, this resulted in enduring relentless teasing that I am not convinced I totally managed to shake off.

'There were other times at school too when friends would tease me about my hearing and although it was always good-natured sometimes I found it difficult. One such incident on a geography field trip resulted in me hitting (not hard) one of my good friends. She being very aware of my dodgy hearing commented that I really should get hearing aids, valid advice really, but not something I was prepared to acknowledge at the time. I'm sure that at the time my confidence took a bit of a knock and inwardly I was feeling scared, but the beauty of avoiding hearing aids was that most of the time I could forget about it. Luckily, because I went to a small school and was surrounded by lots of loud girls who for the most part accepted me as slightly dopey, my grades didn't seem to suffer and I did well in my exams ensuring me a university place.

'It didn't cross my mind to think about how my hearing might have been affected by the lecture theatres and new environments that I was about to encounter as part of university life. In fact, because I had a rather poor attendance rate in my first year of studying I didn't even really notice that I wasn't hearing much if any of what the lecturers were saying.

'It wasn't until the end of my first year that I started to panic again about my hearing. It took me a while to realise that rather than writing down what the lecturer was saying I was just copying their notes from their presentations. Then I realised that when I tried to write down what was being said I couldn't because I couldn't hear the individual words. I don't really remember how it felt at the time but I made the decision then that I was going to get hearing aids.

'At my GP appointment I just said that I wanted a referral and given my history and my age I was given an emergency appointment without hesitation. I think I effectively just ran on auto pilot after that, I didn't think too much about what was happening throughout my testing and then being given my first ever pair of hearing aids having just turned 19.

'Over the years as I have become more open about my hearing, people have often tried to offer solutions to try and cure me. These have varied in method but the result has always been a resounding failure.

The weekend before I was fitted with my first hearing aids I attended a Christian weekend away. I had to leave the trip early on account of collecting my hearing aids, so they were aware of what was happening. They asked if they could pray for my ears in the hope that it might heal me ahead of my appointment the following day. By this point I thought anything was worth a try so they sat me on a chair in the middle of the room some put their hands on my head whilst others prayed around me. The feeling of desperation to fix my hearing and the fear of what was to come plus the hope that perhaps there was a God who was going to help me, resulted in my own belief that this time it might actually work. Waking up the following morning to the familiar stillness felt like waking up at Christmas only to realise it is January and you missed it.

'I had a bit of a love-hate relationship with my first pair of hearing aids. They had ear moulds and because the audiologist thought I might like a funky pair they were also sparkly. A good friend of mine came with me to collect them and was with me during those first moments when I heard with them for the first time. The first sound I remember was the clicking of the door closing then we went outside and I nearly had a heart attack because a car went past and it sounded like a plane taking off.

'It is quite a strange feeling to realise how loud everything is, and sometimes it is actually frustrating. It is tiring too, listening to everything, and I have found that sometimes now even though I can hear what is happening, my brain just switches off when I get tired and everything becomes foreign again.

'When I first started wearing hearing aids my number one priority was that my friends wouldn't find it weird and wouldn't treat me differently. Of course they were fantastic and I think more relieved than

203

anything else. What I didn't completely realise as someone who is hard of hearing is that it can be quite difficult for the people around you. Constantly repeating yourself, being seemingly ignored in the street. Another is that, ironically, I hate repeating myself and by the time I was thinking about getting hearing aids my speech had been quite effected which meant that I was also becoming harder to understand. I have great friends and as far as I know it never put a strain on my relationships with them but it certainly could have.

'Unfortunately even though I have had so many more positive experiences the negative ones are still hard to brush off. More intriguing is that I can actually only remember one time when anyone has ever been negative, which really is a reflection of how our own internal fears about outward perception are normally unfounded. Even though it was only once and it was over four years ago I can still remember where it happened and pretty much what she said which was something along the lines of "that's so weird why would you do that?" It is a shame because it is so insignificant now but it's frustrating that I can't recall the reaction of my friend who was with me when I first left the hospital and how happy she was for me.

'That happened nearly two years before I finally allowed myself to truly think about my hearing and how it might affect the rest of my life. It was then that I struggled the most and was unsure that I would ever be able to cope. I was in my third year at university, I was doing my finals and it was at that point that I started to feel broken beyond repair. Looking back, that does sound melodramatic but at the time all I really felt was despair and I didn't know how to escape from the endless cycle that seemed to consume everything. The reason for my subsequent depression was not just because of my hearing, there were a number

of factors, but it was then that I began to feel all the things that I had avoided since I first started wearing my hearing aids. I was scared of how much more my hearing would deteriorate, I was angry that it had happened to me and I was still embarrassed about what other people might think of me. Worst of all though, I was angry with myself for letting it be such a personal tragedy.

'It took a while to work through it all but I realised that actually it was ok to "grieve" for my ears. I still think it is a terrible word to use for it but it's the best way I can think of to explain it. I let myself feel angry and upset and lost and then I pulled myself together and realised that really it wasn't so bad and in fact now my life was so much easier. I met some very inspiring people who had far more severe hearing loss than my own and I felt a bit foolish that I had let myself get into such a state.

'Hearing loss is such a personal thing and interpreted in so many different ways. Some people I tell say, "Oh no poor you" while others don't understand why it would be a big deal. It is interesting too how people will ask "well how deaf are you?" This is a difficult question to answer because, do they want my audiogram, the results of the words tests I have done, or just a description of what it sounds like? Saying that my hearing is moderate to profound is true but it doesn't really mean much at all in real terms, at least not to me. People also assume that if you don't sign, then you are not that deaf and therefore have no problems coping in the hearing world. This is not always true.

'I went to a hearing conference with a specific focus on children. It was the first time I had ever spent any time with people who communicated predominately in sign language and when they did speak it was hard to follow what they were saying. Many of these people had grown up as part of deaf communities and it was immediately clear (at least from outsider's perspective) that they had an incredibly strong sense of identity and a fantastically supportive network and culture. The conference considered numerous areas and included a variety of workshops, but there was one particular moment that slightly changed my outlook on the hard of hearing world. Someone was giving a talk about hearing in the young, and in general, how some of the consequences must be a sense of isolation and loneliness. From the audience through an interpreter one man explained that actually she was quite wrong. Being part of the deaf community was liberating, inclusive and very far from being lonely. I didn't say it at the time but I disagreed. I had felt very lonely and very isolated. It was in that moment that I wondered for the first time if it was those of us that had some hearing who were the worst off. We are not totally part of the hearing world although we live it and we do not qualify as part of the deaf community because we hear too much. We are stuck in a kind of no man's land where the hearing world assume we are coping fine (or are getting frustrated because we aren't) and we aren't part of the deaf community because we aren't deaf enough. This is just speaking from personal experience, as I am sure there are some who would totally disagree. But there is something about us, in some sort of no man's land, who don't really fit into a category and as a result it seems that there is a real gap in the support, particularly emotionally, that we may benefit from.

'What I have found as a person that sits in this middle zone is that I have had no one to share my experiences with. To talk about getting a hearing aid dome stuck in my ear for two months without realising, or how great it is to sleep at night in nearly total stillness, or how amazing it has been changing hearing aids because of the clarity of the sound *in the new ones. Of course there are many people, including my long suffering family, who I have shared some of these things with, but it isn't the same as talking to someone that actually knows what you are talking about.*

'I decided I wanted to get involved with the UK national hearing charity Action on Hearing Loss (originally RNID). It had become clear to me that we needed to start talking about hearing more and to raise awareness around hearing in the young, particularly for those who were trying to cope in a hearing world and the stigma that might be attached to confronting the problem. I started first as a public speaker talking about my own personal experience. It seemed to make a positive impact on the audiences from the perspective of people that could relate, but also those who couldn't but wanted to understand more. I then decided that I wanted to focus my attention on emotional support for young people making the transition to wearing hearing aids.

'Through research it seemed that nothing of the sort was currently available in the UK, for young people or otherwise. My vision at the time was to create an environment for people to meet with other hearing aid users, either one on one or groups to talk about their fears and concerns but also to share all the positive stories that have come as a result of seeking help. I also felt it important for others to meet people that are getting along just fine in the hearing world, a true reflection of the fact that seeking help isn't a hindrance, it allows for a much better and more rewarding life with very few limitations apart from the ones that you put on yourself.

'I was excited to get this scheme up and running and to reach out to my community. With full support from Action on Hearing Loss we decided to initially focus on London and then grow out depending on

its success. The service was shared with a variety of professionals who would be working with people of the right age bracket, which I had set as 18–25 for the pilot run. We set a date and invited whoever would be interested to come along to the first meeting in which we hoped to help further focus the sort of support that would be most useful. On the day, no one turned up.

'*I had expected it to be hard to draw a crowd and was prepared for the possibility that only one person might come along, partly because the group I was trying to reach are hard to find but also because we have a tendency to not want to talk about it. Even though I wasn't surprised I was incredibly disappointed that I hadn't managed to make it work. It was time to go back to the drawing board and to try to come up with a new strategy that might be more successful. Unfortunately it was also around this time that I was about to go travelling overseas with no idea when I would next be back in the UK. With no one obvious to take over the project, particularly as it was voluntary, the program for now has been put on hold, though I hope now that the idea has been raised it might be resurrected in my absence. What I later learnt, from a lady I met in Australia is that it would be very difficult to draw a crowd to specifically discuss such a topic. We shouldn't focus on the things that we feel either stigmatised by or disabling, but rather on how many things we can do. To bring a group of people together who are hard of hearing for a totally different purpose but with a shared experience is likely to be much more powerful.*

'*Now on my travels and with some time for personal reflection, a chance to consider what I might like to do next and the opportunity to look at my hearing from a different perspective, it has been interesting to both explore more and continue to confront my hearing in terms of what the implications are and how I might be able to make some positive impact for the future.*

'Currently I am spending some time in Australia and I have been so fortunate to have the opportunity to work with Blamey Saunders hears in Melbourne. Both through research for them and as a member of staff for a short time, I have learnt a lot about a world I have so far tried to ignore. They have allowed me to pursue an area that continues to help me make peace with myself and also to understand that I am so much more than what my ears have the capacity to restrict. Through testing not currently available in the UK they have helped me understand the reality of my hearing loss in human terms. Through word tests with Blamey Saunders I was forced to face the severity of my hearing loss. I found it emotionally very hard but it was also a reflection of how incredible my hearing aids are and how lucky I am to not have to cope without them. It was somewhat surreal to be sitting in a room with Professor Blamey who has given so much to the pioneering of Cochlear and also to changing the face of hearing aids that I felt it would be terribly inappropriate to cry. But I did want to.

'Having decided that I would be interested in working in an area that I feel passionately about I have been surprised to find that my most recent experiences have taken me away from wanting to work too closely with hearing over a prolonged period. It is important and it is part of who I am. But it is not who I am. I never want to let it restrict me and it is not what I want people to think of when they think of me. We are what we create ourselves to be and I am a lot more than my hearing.'

Zoe contacted me when she came to Australia, to see what she could learn about services for young people with hearing loss, or deafness. I no longer work with young people's services, but I was really keen to help her. I identified really strongly with travel for a purpose. I've never been all that interested in touring for the sake of it. She ended up volunteering to do research with us. I am continually amazed and grateful to the people who volunteer for us clinical scientists to lend us their ears, and it's a joy to have her working with us. Zoe posed some interesting questions. Is it okay to follow a career that is defined by your deafness?

CHAPTER SIXTEEN

BLAMEY SAUNDERS HEARS — A REVOLUTION IN HEARING AID SERVICE

A legacy of the Churchill fellowship is that I always try to help out other young students travelling. Perhaps as a result of that I have become part of a virtual circle. I reached out to help Zoe but I am the one who has been helped and she is temporarily working with me before her visa runs out. She is now working for me in the hearing aid company I share with Peter Blamey. I feel as though the career adventures that I have had and the skills that I have acquired are now being applied to a very worthwhile cause.

One Saturday afternoon, working long and extra hours for Dynamic Hearing, as usual, Peter and I thought 'There's a better way to do this', so we decided to start a new company, that provided top quality hearing aids that people could set up themselves, and where we, the Doctor and the Professor would supply the hearing aids direct to the end user. We were sure we could see what to do to change people's experience of getting hearing aids. By then we had spent a lot of time in almost every hearing aid company in the world. We wanted the design of the sound processing to be ours, not a mix of our technologies and other people's work. We'd seen too many compromises with our technologies. The owners of Dynamic Hearing wanted to stick with

Dynamic Hearing being a software company, so were not at all interested in our new ideas. We had thought that they would make good sister companies. I thought that the new company should be the one where we could really bring good hearing aid technology, at a really fair cost, to everyone, and also to help people get not only better hearing results but also results that they owned, because they had done the adjustment of their own hearing aids. This would be a company where we supplied self-fit hearing aids, direct to the end user. This would be our company. To this point we had put in many, many hours, and sacrificed our family lives to Venture Capital, and a company that we didn't own. To start the new company, we used our accumulated knowledge of hearing aids and hearing aid technologies to give a fair deal and a good result to people with hearing problems. This would be the company where all the career roles and experiences that I had, along with Peter's vast experience and those things that he and I had jointly done, would come together to start both an audiology clinic and an online hearing aid and audiology company. This is what I am doing today.

Our hearing aids use the technologies that we had developed, and we could use the Internet to take our hearing aids and our audiology anywhere. Our hearing aids resulted, in part, from our cochlear implant experience, and the hearing aids contain technologies that are in the cochlear implants of the Australian implant company at the present time. Thanks to the wonderful developments of the Internet, we can help people set up their hearing aids in their own home, just as if they were in the office with us. Hopefully this new confidence with the Internet encourages our clients to do much more on the Internet. For anyone who is house-bound, it can be a path to substantive conversations and connectedness. We have been able to bring the price of hearing aids down to about half of the going rate for premium end hearing aids. I think my dad would have been proud of what we're doing. We have been able to attract a wonderful team of dedicated people to work with us, including directors of very high calibre.

We have thousands of customers who are very happy. They are taking control of their hearing, like Joanna. We are training young people. We are bringing manufacturing back to Australia. We are integrating our lives with philanthropic work in hearing and in raising awareness about hearing difficulties. And perhaps unexpectedly, but excitingly we are employing some of our family and we are proud of them. I have seen a professional side of my children that I might never have otherwise seen. Running a small company is like having a family and having your own adult children there is very special. A start up company is like having children – personal lives impact everyone, and what we do together, because people care. Like a growing family, every day is different, interpersonal relationships and dynamics play a major part and things keep changing.

We started our new company very quietly, and for a period we both also had very satisfying and exciting day jobs in order to pay our living costs. The Bionic Ear Institute again showed magnificent understanding and helped us by providing excellent facilities at a relatively low rent. They also supplied a collegial and stimulating atmosphere for us in which to get started. After two years of quietly working with customers we launched the business, and our numbers of customers escalated quickly. Blamey Saunders hears supplies world leading hearing aids, coupled with new ways people can set them up themselves at home. People buy the hearing aids from our office, the Internet or by phone and we have supplied hearing aids to people all over Australia, all over the world. We have to have some empathy for very different lifestyles and be prepared to help maintain hearing aids that live in quite extreme environments. Although the hearing aids are undoubtedly excellent, I believe that a big reason for their success is that people set them up themselves. It's quite normal for people to have preferences for particular types of sound: it's not appropriate for everyone to be treated as if they were average, which is pretty much how the traditional methods of hearing aid supply have operated. There is really no such thing as average preferences for listening. I think that listening is based more on the experiences of outliers. Clinicians know that people prefer medical treatments where they are involved in the decision-making. What can be more empowering, in hearing rehabilitation, than setting up your own hearing aid? Hearing aid manufacturers have too long maintained a mystery around hearing aid settings. We have the right technology in our hearing aids and we have made the set up very easy. I can't really imagine inviting someone into my home to adjust the volume of the TV or, worse, the temperature of my shower, so why would I tell you what you want to listen to and how you prefer it to sound. Only you know, and it can be easy to set up.

I really don't understand how audiology and hearing aid companies ended up down this path of fitting hearing aids to the results of the 'soft beep test', or audiogram, and average predictions of what the hearing aid sound output should be. There isn't even agreement on what that prediction should be. Hearing aids need to work well in everyday sound levels, but historically they have been set up to the formulae that I've described. There's a whole industry engaged in developing formulae for this purpose. I don't think they work very well so that you may need to seek a highly qualified professional to tweak the hearing aid away from the formulaic prediction that was first provided, simply to make it acceptable for use.

So, a self-fit hearing aid, where the technology lets you set it up so that you choose what's comfortable (and it stays comfortable) makes a lot of sense. It lets the user take control. It has to be a hearing aid system designed to do this, though, which is why we made one. We set out to have hearing aids that are so smart that you can set them up yourself, saving time and money, but with a support system using the Internet, so people can have help if they want. Australia is big. I sometimes need to remind myself that working in Melbourne and supplying technology and hearing aids to people in Perth is not unlike being in London and supplying technology to Vladivostok. But because Australia has big distances to deal with, we are accustomed to finding innovative solutions for the problem. Australia developed the School of the Air and pioneered the Flying Doctor service. Now Australia has a hearing aid and remote service audiology company, working across the whole of Australia and expanding work across the world. The tyranny of distance is something we, in Australia, have to overcome: perhaps it helps make us innovative and requires us to find new solutions to overcome the problems.

With Peter Blamey, and the rest of my team, I am pioneering the hearing aid delivery model of the future. You, the hearing aid user needn't go out of the house. We've invented hearing aids that people can set up with their smart phone, without an audiologist, although I have a commitment to complete service if someone wants that. We've built a model where the hearing test is done at home, the hearing aid and self-fit system is delivered to home, and the client sets it up themselves, with help, according to their preference. We supply as much or as little help as the customer wants. With or without help, It's the client's choice. We can set up the hearing aids for our client over the Internet, just as if they were in our hearing clinic, or we can just give them some encouragement as they do it themselves. I prefer people to set the hearing aids up for themselves because to get the best possible results only they truly know what they want to hear. Also, once the user has the ability to easily tweak the settings of their hearing aids at home, they can readjust as often as they wish as their understanding of their new 'hearing' world grows, and without multiple audiologist visits. Not everyone has the imagination or knowledge to see why this approach should, and does, work. Perhaps I am naïve and it is actually competitive interest that drives the apparent lack of comprehension of the obvious? At times I have had to be thick skinned; you can't change an industry, without creating some disgruntled people in the industry. Being a disruptive innovator is tough: but I really only care about my clients, and people with hearing problems. I am not known as 'The Hearing Lady' at Rotary for nothing.

I had to train a 'behind the scenes' team at Blamey Saunders to help me run the service. This means we can supply a much bigger range of expert help than a single local audiologist. We, like many people who are 'Firsts', have taken the brunt of the heat of discontent and opposition from the incumbents in the industry. But the path I am on is rewarding and exciting. When I was working with deaf children in the early 1970s I could not have imagined that we would be supplying hearing aids with mini computers over the Internet. In the course of researching the business model for Blamey Saunders, I found that most people like to compare their own hearing with that of other people. People like to do 'a test' to confirm their beliefs about their hearing, or even to refute what other people have observed. I used our own Blamey Saunders Speech Perception Test (SPT) to let about 20 people test their own hearing, at a Rotary Club in Dubbo recently. Everyone who took the test already had a very realistic view of their hearing ability, but they wanted 'A Test' to confirm it. Research shows that people who have acquired hearing loss during their life know that they have hearing problems. A study carried out in Finland showed that the answer to the question, 'Do I have hearing difficulties?' if honestly answered was a very good test of hearing. But for some reason people don't trust their own judgement. Perhaps they don't want to know. Perhaps they have been conditioned to need an 'expert' to pronounce on their 'ailment'. So, Peter Blamey invented a new test of hearing (The SPT) based on the work of George Miller and Patricia Nicely, which tells you which sounds of speech you can hear well and which sounds of speech you have trouble hearing. Blamey Saunders owns the test, but we want this to be available to everyone as a community tool. So we put it online and anyone with a computer, computer speakers, or headphones and an Internet connection can do the tests at home and can get their results immediately, at no cost. We can use those results to set up our hearing aids and post them out. The person who has done the test can do the test again then with their new hearing aids on to make sure that they are benefiting from the aids. So going back to my comparison with the School of the Air, our customers can, while staying at home, test their hearing, order their hearing aids and then adjust them, while saving time, money and inconvenience and getting a top quality result because they've done it for themselves. Needless to say, I'm not particularly popular with the people who currently sell hearing aids. However, I am keen that audiologists start to value once again their skills in helping people to adjust to hearing aids, listen again and relearn good communication skills. While I am never likely to be popular with resellers of hearing aids in the current style of audiological service, I know I'm a good audiologist and we have a clinic where people who want personal face-to-face services can come for advice and where I have students to supervise to ensure that good skills are passed on. I am also keen that we continue to do world-class research on ways to test hearing and on ways to help people make the most of their hearing. We will also continue to speak to the community to raise awareness of the importance of acting on hearing difficulties, and we are doing that in some innovative ways, including the production of *The Sound of Waves*.

My educational foundation in quantum physics taught me to be open minded about solutions. I think I am good at asking questions, seeing a need, pursuing a cause and I know I am good at finding very clever people to help pursue the causes. We are making a real and positive difference by improving hearing for those in need. I wish these solutions had been here in the early 1970s to help the children I worked with then. The Internet is changing the way health care is practiced throughout the world and Australia is catching up. Health care planners recognize the important health benefits of more home based care, more self-management, and more autonomy for both urban and rural populations. It's economically essential for Australia to relieve the growing financial pressures on hospitals and face-to-face health delivery services. We have had some help from both the Victorian and the Federal Government to ensure that our systems are easy to use, and our new programming system is helping to build manufacturing capability in Australia.

Health care experts in Australia agree that, in many areas of health care, Tele-health technology is already available for more home-based care and more efficient management of chronic health conditions. Tele-health (remote health, e-health) addresses the collection and/or exchange of information electronically between doctors, allied health professionals, and patients in both synchronous and asynchronous modes. Experts also recognise that change management is needed to help established health practitioners to change their approach, but recent graduates (including audiologists) can be described as digitally naive, and should be poised to embrace the opportunities that technology enhanced healthcare can effect.

Research shows that Tele-health can actually enhance quality of care by better supporting chronic disease management, application of best practices, while visit based care in healthcare practices and institutions is the most expensive form of care delivery. By extending the healthcare system using other communication and collaboration technologies and making the best use of all clinicians and staff in the healthcare system, we can develop a scalable healthcare system that will be a model care delivery system for the future.

Globally, there are no clear trends as to which areas of healthcare will become the leaders in tele-health, and they are likely to be driven by a combination of consumer needs and the most innovative companies. In my role with Rotary International to help address hearing loss issues worldwide, I have become aware, from community questions that these issues are not going to be solved with the model of audiological care that has been common for the last 25 years. It is too labour intensive and too expensive even for developed countries.

My company, Blamey Saunders is leading in remote hearing aid provision and tele-audiology in Australia. We have 20 people, including audiologists, scientists, engineers, technicians and support staff and we are excited about our combined clinic and Tele-audiology practice. The Hearing CRC in Australia have published a summary on their website, Hearnet, about Cochlear Ltd's ongoing studies in cochlear implant tele-practice, and their results show that people are very satisfied with the process of hearing care at home. It's not really surprising that room service is satisfactory. A Masters of Audiology student, at the University of Auckland, Erin Keach, found a similar level of high satisfaction, when people set up their own hearing aids.

Tele-health services are currently coming into use in the rural and remote sector, which also provides for indigenous communities in Australia. Now that web-based remote and rural services have been established in the private sector, the Government has an opportunity to integrate this into their established service. This would enable delivery of services to meet the extraordinary demand that will occur as people become more aware of the importance of using hearing aids. Audiologists' work will become more valued as we become more effective, help more people remotely, and continue working face-to-face with the most challenging part of our caseload. As audiologists with face-to-face clinical practices, we will probably be busier than ever, and even more challenged. This is because more accessible service models will increase the awareness of hearing aid benefit, and take up the majority of the primary level hearing care. From this enlarged population of hearing aid users, an increased number of complex cases will emerge, requiring face-to-face consultation. Whilst there are many indicators of client complexity, it is well recognised that this doesn't always emerge at first encounter. Indeed, some don't emerge until well down the track, or circumstances and client needs change. Changes in needs or circumstances present a particular challenge for our remote and rural communities, but the tele-health model will help to identify these cases and provide appropriate treatment earlier.

Increasingly, the Internet is becoming an essential service for the elderly. It is the pivotal component of home-based care, enabling not just rehabilitation and health care delivery, but also being a conduit to information and access to outside services such as grocery shopping, and to social interaction. U.S. data show that older Internet users use the Internet for accessing information, and the Internet is the primary source of information for 45 to 65 year olds today in Australia. In 2013, the fastest adoption of social networks took place with people 74 years of age or older. This makes it critical that we recognise current trends, and guide people with hearing loss, who are relying on the Internet for information. As clinicians interested in the wellbeing of our clients, our approach should be rigorous in providing information on purchasing hearing aids. It is our community of audiologists who should be helping readers understand that there is a huge difference in a self-fit hearing aid with audiologist guided tele-health service support and aftercare, and a hearing aid or AID, of 'uncertain provenance' on e-bay. We should be helping our clients to discriminate and choose effective solutions. As clinicians, we should welcome the new era, and the increased opportunity to be valued tertiary care professionals and experts, rather than 'hearing aid sales guys'. Tele-health will give audiologists a renewed opportunity to be valued and remunerated as clinicians using modern methods.

Similar findings have been reported for hearing aids, with appropriate technology and processes, including availability of support. Tele-practice makes the clinician more available – you are only an email away. Tele-practice provides clients the opportunity to be instantly in contact with a team of experts. My personal experience as a leader of a remote hearing aid fitting company, which supplies self-fit hearing aids, is that maintaining a strong research and community outreach focus is extremely important. It is personally satisfying seeing a team of audiologists leading support staff and working with people remotely all over Australia. One day you are helping someone on an oil rig, and the next day a farmer; this can be obvious from the hearing aids coming in for maintenance, that reflect the different environments they have been exposed to.

The key people in our company are the audiologists. Being leaders in Tele-audiology has enabled us to develop a strong research database, to evaluate the efficacy of solutions, and to constantly improve our systems and outcomes. There is a reduction in cost of travel and reduction of barriers to care. Our collective goal, as audiologists, is surely a combined, remote and face-to-face approach to care. This allows for respect of individual preferences, circumstances and complexity.

Tele-health is not just a traditional model of care, conducted by video conference. Tele-health is doing things differently. The Cochlear example and my company are examples of 'doing it differently' to achieve client centred and client empowered care.

The Blamey Saunders hears self fit hearing aid system is such good technology that people experience excellent results and comprises product at about one third of the cost of other premium quality hearing aids. This is different to the traditional market, we needed to think hard how to approach it.

The hearing aid market is traditionally driven through audiologist or hearing aid dispenser as the main sales channels. The industry is highly vertically integrated and many audiologists are predominantly employed in sales roles. The hearing aids are typically priced according to the number of enabled features. It is a retail sector where the product has been traditionally associated with aging, and that to get hearing aids have been seen as an admission of aging. The existing business model focuses on identifying those people whose hearing is severely impaired and charging them a great deal to re-instate some level of hearing.

We wanted to use the advanced technology and our business process vision to change this, and to be disruptive in the market. The challenges were many. We employed design thinking in order to overcome a perception that the business might be seen just as an online business selling hearing aids directly to the end customer, at a reduced price, and, competing on price against this firmly entrenched, traditional retail model. We wanted to convey that, done properly, a business that provides care at home could be better than traditional models.

In the traditional model, clients are often drawn into the sales funnel by the offer of free hearing tests. The sales 'prospects' are then offered hearing aids where the product price is bundled with a service cost and a substantial cost multiple then applied. The Blamey Saunders hears model uses high quality sound processing that works in all environments, and a simplified hearing aid personalisation process. We achieved our initial growth with strong exposure of the unique features of the product, its origins and the team. The next phase of growth came through word-of-mouth recommendations as our marketing story consolidated, but they needed a strong design strategy to achieve their goal of not only gaining a significant share of the market but also growing the market.

To communicate our story, we partnered with a design company, and used the process of Strategic Design Thinking – this is a relatively new term that indicated in communicating key messages about a company, you needed to work with the bigger picture. My goal was to apply Design Thinking, to develop a strategy where we could communicate to our potential clients and customers that they would become empowered by taking control of their hearing, and that this is an important health message. I also wanted to communicate that they would be purchasing from a leading research and clinical team. I wanted my whole team to have strong and greater clarity of purpose. I wanted them to understand what we do, why we do it and for us to work together to find the best ways to do it. The move into the area of Design Thinking was another career first, but one which I have thoroughly enjoyed. Scientists don't have a reputation for good communication. The Design Thinking was going to strengthen our sense of purpose, and communication.

I have one more puzzle. People often ask me about the 'Stigma' of hearing aids. I am so focused on trying to help people get timely access to hearing aids that I tend to forget that some people don't want them. Is there a stigma to hearing aids? Or is there a stigma of 'Old Age'. Older people have more commonly used hearing aids partly because the community has not been widely informed of the importance of getting on with the uptake of hearing aids as soon as possible after starting to have some difficulty hearing clearly. Otherwise there would be lots more people donning hearing aids at about the same time as they start using glasses. If in fact, people don't wear hearing aids because they make them look old: then the stigma is about aging, not about hearing aids. It's not using hearing aids that make you look old, its 'not using' hearing aids that indeed accelerates aging. We have brought down the price of hearing aids extensively, but this is not enough to help many of the people around the world who don't have access to any solutions. I've recently become involved in the Rotary action group on hearing. This has brought home to me that the challenge we are facing is to help more than 350 million people around the world who have hearing loss, but no access to hearing aids. I will keep encouraging people who have access to hearing aids to get them, to use them and to live life to the full. In the Western world, and developed world, most of the people who would benefit from hearing aids don't get them or don't use them, even though we know that untreated hearing loss leads to a massive reduction in quality of life. This might be through simple isolation, which may be due to the downstream problems of depression, unemployment, or reduced cognitive function. People are worried about the cosmetics and the cost. I think we have helped with both. But I continue to do a lot of education to the general public on the importance of taking early action with hearing loss and getting on with using hearing aids.

CHAPTER SEVENTEEN

TO HEAR OR NOT TO HEAR: THAT WASN'T A QUESTION...

Let's listen to Louise's story.

ON LOSING HEARING

'To me, the world of sound was almost everything. From a young age, playing the piano and singing in the school choir were sources of great joy to me. Creating and hearing the richness of notes in their infinite possibilities was the ultimate in creative expression. Listening to music ranging from classical to rock, it brought a light to my soul. Did I think I had good hearing? Of course I did. I must have. When I was young I could remember pointing the locations of "silent" alarms as I accompanied my mum to jewellery stores, those set supposedly to high frequencies inaudible to the human ear. My opinion in music was valued. I was the first female rock DJ for my university's radio station during the coveted 4–5 Friday afternoon time slot. I knew what I was doing because I could hear what was going on.

'Did I know when I first started losing my hearing or why? No, I did not. I suspect it was from going to rock concerts and standing close to the massive speakers, but I can't be sure. But I do remember starting to notice in my mid-40s that when I went to parties and luncheons where there were a lot of people talking around me, I often couldn't understand what someone standing near me and talking to me was saying. I have to also admit I noticed that other people were not having any trouble understanding each other in these settings where I was struggling. I noticed it but I also dismissed it as not meaning anything. I had fabulous hearing after all. There was no issue in my mind. No problem at all.

'I do remember by the time I was 50 I began to feel uncomfortable in groups of people where there were multiple conversations going on. I was vaguely aware that I was always struggling to maintain a dialogue with someone I was very close to but was quick to dismiss this as meaning anything. Endlessly asking someone to repeat what they had just said and then still not understand it. Pretending to follow a conversation when I didn't have a clue what they were saying. I cupped my ear to capture more noise. These were strategies I adopted to cope with noisy social situations. But it wasn't fun and at best I was only picking up on every third word. I remember feeling isolated and frustrated that I wasn't able to connect with the people around me. Now at night, when there was supposed silence all around me, I could hear a roaring in my ears, I noticed when I was really tired it was particularly loud. What was this from? What was this noise? I never investigated what I later learned was tinnitus, a common complaint for those experiencing hearing loss. All of this was so gradual, that I just didn't connect the dots. All the signs were there, I just didn't look at them.

'Without realising what I was doing, I began avoiding these social gatherings where I had to hear more than one voice at a time. If friends wanted to get together, I made a point of seeing them solo. How else did it affect me? My husband and my daughter used to complain that I would turn on the TV too loud. I thought they were being precious. The sound on the new TV just wasn't as good as the old TV. And as for music, well, I just turned the speakers up in the car full volume.

'My eyes were opened to the fact that I indeed did have a hearing loss, through a freak accident in which my left eardrum was punctured. I was washing my husband's car in the carport that was right next to a small garden bed filled with sword ferns. When I leant over to wash the car's undercarriage, I somehow turned my head to the perfect wrong position so that a sword fern spike went through my ear and perforated the ear drum so I could no longer hear at all through my left ear. A quick trip to the doctor reassured me that my hearing would go back to normal once the perforation healed itself in a few weeks. I become very conscious of what I was hearing and not hearing, and recognised that I simply could not hear as well as I used to. My doctor sent me to an audiologist where I underwent the standard hearing "beep" test. My second appointment with the audiologist to get the results was very revealing.

"I have some good news and some bad news," he told me. "Which do you want first?"

"The good news," I said.

"Your eardrum has completely repaired itself and it is infection free."

"So – there is bad news?" I wondered out loud.

"You have significant hearing loss in both ears, and this is not related in any way to your punctured eardrum," the audiologist told me.

I was genuinely astonished.

"No, I don't," I told him.

"Yes, you do," he replied.

"No, I don't. I pushed the buzzer every time I heard a sound."

"You missed the sounds at the higher frequencies," he told me.

"Why? Will my hearing come back?"

"We cannot be certain but most likely it was from overexposure to a series of loud noises. And no, your hearing will not revert to normal hearing."

'I still couldn't believe it. But upon returning home a quick discussion with my husband confirmed what the audiologist was telling me. My husband told me I was always insisting on having the TV and car radio at almost an intolerably loud volume. So I now knew what my reality was. I did not have great hearing or even good hearing for that matter. This meant that I could no longer hear music the way I once did. But as far as I was concerned, that was the end-of-story. I was not what you would call, a "happy camper" to have this new knowledge. Wearing hearing aids was not going to be an option for me. I wasn't going to be one of "those people" (whatever that meant) who wore them because not only was I too young to need them (again whatever that meant) but I somehow imagined that music would now sound like an early recording – tinny, reedy and not very true to what was being played. I loved music and how it made me feel. I wasn't going to have it ruined by what I was sure was inferior sound quality. Nope, I wasn't going to do anything about this.'

ON GETTING HEARING AIDS

'So I was stubborn and chose to ignore what I now knew for certain was the truth. The trouble was the truth in a way did set me free but to *start with not in a good way. All those parties and lunches with friends with noisy backgrounds became completely intolerable. I could "see" that I really couldn't hear like my friends could and I became very self-conscious that my "hearing" strategies were not working as well as I pretended they were. None of this was fair. But what should I do? What did I do? For a year, I chose to do nothing. I simply gritted my teeth, ignored my husband and daughter's complaints about how loud the TV was being played and spoke to no one about what I was going through.*

'As a freak accident enlightened me to my hearing loss, a moment of serendipity put me on the path of meeting Elaine Saunders and getting hearing aids. At this time, I was accompanying my young daughter to an Anglican church with a reasonable sized congregation. They needed volunteers to teach the various groups in their Sunday school. I put my hand up to help and by chance was paired with Elaine's daughter Amy to oversee one group of students. Amy and I got on very well and I remember thinking although she was 15, she brought to the table some remarkably astute and highly relevant strategies and ideas to each of our students. As we grew to know each other, I remember her mentioning in passing that her mother was the CEO of hearing research facility Dynamic Hearing. How interesting. What were the odds? I had been a member of this church for years and never met or heard of her mum and I seriously doubt if I hadn't decided to help out at their Sunday school and just happen to have her daughter as my assistant that I would have. Was this someone I could at least ask what my options were? I didn't know and found myself too embarrassed to bring it up. But the struggle of trying to understand what other people were saying had reached the point I knew I had to swallow my pride as I was getting tired of saying "What?" 30–40 times a day.

'So I met with Elaine. She later told me I was clearly very angry about not having great hearing. She very patiently heard me out – all my frustrations about the situation I was in and all my misconceptions about how awful wearing hearing aids would be – not to mention what poor sound quality they would produce. (This thinking in hindsight somehow bemuses me as I had never actually tried them or spoken to anyone who wore them.)

'I am convinced if it hadn't been for Elaine; it may have been years before I did anything about my hearing. She invited me to her research facility Dynamic Hearing to trial a range of hearing aids, gently suggesting I explore my options. I remember she stressed she wasn't concerned with what hearing aids brand I selected if I chose to purchase a pair. She was more concerned that I was happy with sound. And yes, hearing aids were now designed to cater to music lovers with a special programme to best capture and enhance the sound quality of each note. She allayed my fears about the whole experience enough to accept it was time to be open-minded – I really wasn't too young, old or whatever to do something about this. This is the only approach that would have worked for me; I wasn't open-minded enough at this point to respond to a company pushing their brand. It was time to give it a go.

'Fast forward to the day when I tried my first hearing aids on. I had been through the testing of my hearing and the discussions of what my concerns were with the audiologist Elaine had arranged for me to see. I put them on – tucking the tiny tube into each ear and looping the small casing that housed the hearing aid's electronics behind my ear, closed the battery case, heard the "beeps" that the audiologist told me I would hear when the hearing aids turned on, and listened.

I will never forget this moment. I was stunned. I honestly did not know just what I had been missing. Outside, I heard a car in the alleyway, its wheels spinning making a high pitch sound as they turned. And then there was a splash as the car went through a puddle – a sound that wasn't muted. It was a sound with all richness of sparkling diamonds – something I hadn't heard in years. I clapped my hand over my mouth and I think I gasped.

"What is going on?" The audiologist was speaking to me. Her words were so clear!?! "Quick, tell me," she said.

"Do you mean to tell me that everyone can hear what I am hearing now?" I asked her.

"What do you hear?" Her words! I understood them without hearing aids but now there was fullness in the consonants.

"Yes," she replied when I told her what I was experiencing. "Everyone with normal hearing can hear what you are hearing now.'

"Are you sure you haven't just turned up some amplifier so it is louder than normal?" I asked.

She just laughed. "Actually, I have set the hearing programme slightly under what would be normal hearing so you have some time to adjust to all the new sounds."

'And there were so many, it was wonderful and astounding to say the least. Walking on a tiled floor, a door closing, someone sneezing – these were sounds I had always been able to hear. But now, there was richness, a three dimensionality to the quality. And all those voices I struggled to understand – I knew what people were saying, but intriguing was the sounds I could hear that I simply had lost the ability to hear. The beep of a phone, the trickle of water running or the sounds coming from another room. I hadn't known what I didn't hear.

'And music! The joy of it all! I never did lose my love of it but now that the richness in the texture of each note connected to each other is accessible to me again I experience it in the fullness that is available to those who have normal hearing. To go to hear a live symphony, to turn on the radio and experience the roundness of each sound each artist has chosen to produce. Words fail me. The closest analogy I can come up with is equating hearing with vision. Imagine living in a world where it is deep twilight and the many colours of the rainbow spectrum are deeply muted; only you don't know you can't see what everyone else can. Getting hearing aids is like having someone turn on the lights again for you.

'And it wasn't till Elaine asked me to write this that I wondered if I would have found the same joy in dancing if I hadn't chosen to do something about my hearing, a passion that I discovered several years after getting my first hearing aids.'

ON BECOMING AN AMAZING DANCER

'Elaine has asked me to talk about my journey to becoming the dancer I am today. I guess I should start by saying that I have never taken on any new venture in my life half-heartedly. Everyone has a different approach to living their life and I am one of those boots and all people. Having said that, I don't think I have ever done anything that I loved as much as I love dancing.

'A cold call on the telephone from a telemarketer gave me three free private dance lessons at a social dance studio, and that is all it took. Within a matter of weeks, I was a regular fixture at this new home away from home as I earnestly worked with other fellow students to learn *everything I could about ballroom and Latin dancing. This studio was wonderful for giving everyone the opportunity to express themselves in a showcase format. It was here that I was able to explore telling a story through using music as the backdrop. I also learned basic technique of eight dances: the waltz, foxtrot, tango, quickstep, rumba, cha cha cha, samba and the swing.*

'But while everyone around me seemed to be content with learning a seemingly infinite variety of step combinations, after several years I realised that this simply was not enough for me. I was initially reluctant to let anyone know that I had hearing difficulties and I compounded the problem by not wearing my hearing aids on any occasion where I had to wear my hair back or up – thereby increasing the chances of people seeing them. Again, in retrospect – what difference did that really make? They didn't look that noticeable. But the sad thing was that I was still not comfortable with anyone knowing that I had trouble hearing. Never mind the fact that when I did start telling people, it was not uncommon for them to say, "Oh, that's why it seemed like you used to ignore me. I said something to you once, and you walked by me like you didn't even know I was there!" (I probably didn't.)

'But back to my story, dance involves the ability to count and dance to the beat of the music and what I was hearing now involved much more than just step patterns as guided by my teacher's around the floor. I really wanted to learn to dance in the full sense of the word – to use my body to express all the stories that music evokes. And they seemed endless, another new story for every song. There was so much more that I needed to learn well beyond the social arena. I had become a bit of an identity at this studio, not being one to be shy about dancing or what I was looking for but all the same, it came as a bit of a surprise to most

except for my closest friends when I left the studio to go to Space – a dance centre for professionals, dance students and just about anyone who wanted to learn the nitty gritty about dance. I somehow talked my way into a Latin American dance troupe – most of them being half my age and three times my skill level at that time.

"It is up to the group", the dance choreographer and leader told me flatly, "If they don't want you, I'm sorry, you won't be able to join."

'For whatever reason, those 11 amazing dancers welcomed me to their fold and this began a journey to learning how to dance using my whole body, mind and spirit. I was no longer given words of encouragement by my new teacher, it was all tough love. Sink or swim. If it hadn't been for the patience of some of the troupe members during our extra practice time, I am not sure how I would have made it to performance day several months later, much less get the first compliment from my dance teacher, "I have never seen you dance that well."

'That was almost two years ago, and this troupe has since disbanded after several performances, each going our own way in the dance world. To this day, though, we stay in touch, some of us on a weekly basis, to encourage, support and experience each other's efforts and skills on the dance floor.

'I seemed to have collected a group of friends who come and watch me perform – every chance they get. Why? I know what they say about me. They tell me they can see the love I have for dance, the drive. They tell me I have an amazing spirit and that I am an inspiration. I really don't see it that way. I am just trying to do the best with what I have. I started later in life, but that has given me the freedom to really bring to life all those stories for all that music I can know here. I am not inspirational, but I think people like Elaine Saunders are – those who are bringing to life a vision that is more than just self-expression. They are truly helping other people through bettering their quality of life. A quote attributed to Helen Keller – a remarkable woman who grew up deaf and blind and in her early years, dumb in a time there was virtually no support for such people best addresses their approach to life:

> "No pessimist ever conquered the stars, or sailed to an unchartered land or opened a new heaven to the human spirit."

'I think I am able to do the things I do in dance today, partly because she showed me the door to the wonderful world of sound where my heart is.'

CHAPTER EIGHTEEN

People hearing without listening

Have you ever been told that you're not listening? I suspect most people have been told that at some time or another. So what is listening? Is it the same as hearing? No it's not.

We use our hearing to make sense of the world around us and to communicate, but it's listening that makes sense of the hearing. We have filters in our ears to help hear in noise. We have listening filters in our brain to help attend to what we think is important. Getting sound in, using hearing aids helps us to keep the listening filters in our brain in better shape. But we still need to practice.

It's a good idea to take time to listen to the sounds around you. Go somewhere quiet, or somewhere that you think is quiet, and then attend and listen to the sounds that you can hear. Try to identify the sound that is furthest away. Try and listen for a new sound. Can you identify all the sounds that you can hear? Share this listening experience with someone else. I gave this advice in a talk once and someone in the audience said that she often went to the end of the garden with her granddaughter just to sit and listen. I thought that was a lovely thing to do and she is helping her granddaughter learn to listen.

Listening involves more than just our ears. We have four engines to use for hearing and listening – two eyes and two ears. The use of all four engines is a skill that's well developed by the time we are six months old. We should continue to use this skill. If you are listening to someone talk, it's much nicer for the speaker if you're looking at them. It's an important part of active listening, and sets the scene for a good communication interaction. Most people's faces give away a lot of information, this is not irrelevant as our brain uses facial expressions to set context for what it could hear. Body language is a strategy to help make listening a little bit easier. As we get older. Some of the processes that we use in hearing and listening slow down or deteriorate. That makes it especially important not just to use hearing aids, but also to engage our eyes and our brain as fully as possible in the listening process. It's kind of a way of keeping fit. I think its easier than working out.

'Listening can make the difference between a longer career and a shorter one', so wrote Bernard Ferrari, in a recent McKinsey Quarterly magazine. Good listening means attending to and understanding the information presented. This might involve asking a lot of questions. Whether you are in a business meeting or a restaurant, asking questions can be a good way to make sure you have understood. It is also another positive reinforcement to the speaker that you are listening.

If you decide to get hearing aids, firstly, make sure they are good ones. There is a huge difference between a low quality hearing aid and a good hearing aid. It's a great shame that people talk about hearing aids collectively as if they are all the same: they are not, which is why I have spent my life working towards excellent hearing aids. Then when you have the hearing aids, you have to use them, preferably all the time. I think this should be a really positive experience so I put together a few ideas, over the next few pages, of how to spend the first ten days with your hearing aids. If you use them all the time, you are on the right path to hearing fitness. Stay on this path, and you will always have a hearing solution. You are also more likely to stay in better brain shape. You have taken the first step in your hearing fitness plan.

Now it's important to use your new ears well to fine-tune your listening skills. If you have automatic, adaptive directional microphones, they will help you in background noise, and you will be able to hear speech sounds better, if you use them properly. To get advantage from them, you need to use them optimally. You need to keep your head turned to the speaker of interest – not just the eyes, but your head.

There's a book I like called *The One Percent Principle,* written by Tom O'Neil: his message is that small things can get great results. 'You can make a huge difference in your world if you choose, one percent at a time.' I've applied this to getting a good, positive start with hearing aids.

DAY 1

Set up your new hearing aids so they're set at your listening comfort levels. Unpack the drying jar, so it's ready to use tonight. Now put on the hearing aids and do something that you really enjoy. Make today the first day of the next stage of your hearing and listening life and celebrate it. If you're at work, maybe you can go out to lunch today.

Keep your hearing aids on all day if you can.

Your ear canal is lined with very sensitive skin. If the hearing aids feel a bit itchy, don't worry about it, and still try to keep them in for much of the day. The itchy feeling will go away. At the end of the day, if you feel you'd like to take the hearing aid out, that's okay. If the itchy feeling doesn't go away within about three days, then, it's possible that you have some underlying skin irritation, and you should get it medically checked.

Today is the day to start good habits with your new hearing aids.

When you take off your hearing aids, open the battery door fully, to turn them off. Put them in the drying jar for the night. This is especially important if you live somewhere humid.

DAY 2

If you've got time to have another day of doing something you really enjoy again, then do that, but if it's back to normal routine, then try to incorporate some special listening activities in your day. Can you hear new sounds? Can you recognise all the sounds you are hearing? The hearing aids probably sound great. If there is less bass sound than you expected, your hearing system will soon learn to interpret the treble sound again. It just means the brain has forgotten it.

Today, enjoy wearing your new hearing all day. You might still prefer to take them off in the evening and don't worry if you do.

You may be forgetting that you are wearing them by now, but if you are one of the people for whom they still feel a bit new, then that's OK too.

DAY 3

Today you are going to listen to more new sounds. Listen to the rhythm of the sounds. If you like television or radio then listen to a program you like, and enjoy hearing more. Good hearing aids will automatically adjust to make sounds audible and comfortable all the time, so the TV should be at a comfortable volume.

Choose some sounds in your house, or your work place that sound a bit similar. Learn to tell the difference between them.

If you can go with a friend somewhere where there are lots of people talking, practice listening to them against other voices. The hearing aids will help you as long as your head is turned to the speaker. Practice good, attentive listening strategies.

DAY 4

You probably won't need new batteries yet, but you might like to check that you are comfortable changing the hearing aid batteries today.

This isn't difficult but if your hands are a bit unsteady then work on a nice clear table. Open the battery compartment; take out the old battery; take a new battery out of the pack; put it in the battery compartment, paper side up; peel off the paper; shut the compartment; that's all! The new one will last for about a week, but it's a good idea to keep a spare with you, in case it runs out at an inconvenient moment.

Today, keep the hearing aids on until you retire for the night. Enjoy the sharpness of sounds and the greater clarity it brings.

DAY 5

You are probably good at slipping the hearing aids on or off by now. If you aren't, don't worry, but take some time to practice. Either use a mirror, or have someone help you. If you wear earrings, make sure you are able to get the hearing aids on and off without them getting tangled. You'll find a way that suits you. Once you've put the hearing aids on, spend the rest of the day enjoying them. Can you find and recognise some new sounds today?

DAY 6

Today have a go at a quick service of your hearing aid. It is a good idea to wipe the ear tip with an alcohol wipe or damp tissue before you put it in each day (just like one cleans glasses). Earwax can commonly block the speaker. To make sure it's all clear, take off the tip; clean it or replace it, and then change the wax stop. That's the little white piece at the edge of the speaker. Work on a flat surface, and perhaps on a dark cloth. Take your time. Being able to do this will give you a lot of confidence in maintaining your hearing aids.

Today listen around you to more sounds and see if you can tell which ones are furthest away. You will have a bigger hearing range now, so it is good practice to listen to sounds and see if you can identify which ones are from a distance.

DAY 7

Have you been into a place where there are a lot of people talking yet? If not, try today. Make sure you turn your head to look directly at the person you want to listen to. This is really important. Don't just turn your eyes to them – turn your head to face them, so that the directional microphones are activated and give you some help. The combination of the directional microphones and watching the speaker's face will be a big help to you.

DAY 8

Hopefully you are using your hearing aids fully now, and you are enjoying the experience. You might not get so tired, as you won't have to concentrate so hard to hear.

You've had hearing aids for a week now, so make a few notes about all the new sounds and experiences you've had. If there was anything you didn't like, have a think about 'Why'. Perhaps you had forgotten about some sounds that are a bit noisy.

Perhaps your voice doesn't sound as nice as you remember it, or perhaps your car is noisier than you thought; perhaps there are household sounds you don't like very much. It's normal life to have sounds that you don't like. Alternatively you can try to find something that you do after all like about the sound.

DAY 9

A few people still find it hard to hear clearly with even the best hearing aids. This is because there are other things wrong in the hearing and listening system, and listening in noise is not just a problem of detecting sounds. There are lots of different reasons, but the answer is the same for all of them, practice, practice and more practice.

Auditory memory: there are some things you can practice.

Ask a friend to recite three numbers to you. Then recite them back, in reverse order. When you can do three, do four. Ask a friend to read a passage of three sentences. When they have finished, tell them the first and the last word of the passage.

Music training: try a music-training program, such as theta music. It's free, and there is scientific evidence that music training helps listening skills.

DAY 10

Now it's time to get serious. You are about to enter the path to being an expert listener. Efficient listening is at least partly about skill. Of course, you need to be able to hear – that's why you have new hearing aids.

In general, processes of aging make it harder to hear in background noise, but the good news is that there are things we can do.

Generally, as we get older:

- The hearing system processes speech more slowly. This affects temporal coding of sound.
- There is reduced working auditory memory ability (this is not the same as having memory lapses). Think of it as the RAM in your computer. This affects our ability to hold complex sound patterns in memory. This skill is important as your auditory memory makes it possible for you to recognise words.
- Hearing deteriorates in the sense organ of hearing, reducing our ability to sort out individual frequencies.
- Reduced ability to fuse the inputs from two ears, this is called binaural fusion, and helps us hear in noise.

Now the good news:

- As we get older, we acquire a lot of hearing and listening practice and can use this to hear and listen well.

- We gain social experience, linguistic knowledge, lip reading and facial expression reading ability. We use all of this, and can practice some of it.

So now that you have become a hearing aid user, you can practice all these other things too, to become a Power Hearing Aid User. I like to give people some general hints too: don't be afraid to ask people to talk a little more slowly, and to face you. They probably won't mind, and anyway, it's good communication training for them. Don't worry if you get tired. That's normal as you adjust. When you are comfortable with your hearing aids, you should find life less tiring than before you got them. Try to get the people you live with and work with to practice better communication habits. Get rid of reverberant surfaces and unwanted noise where you can. Blamey Saunders hears was founded to be a company for social good. I believe you don't have to be in a developing country to do this. Our prices are low; our service is high, and we support a number of philanthropic projects and a lot of community education with our time.

Whilst we are a 'for profit' company every member of my team knows what we do and why. They understand that our goal is to help as many people as possible, people with hearing difficulties. I have helped people in their 30s and 40s who otherwise couldn't afford quality hearing aids. I have helped people on remote farms who are many hours drive from the nearest audiology service. Every aspect of our care is client focused. If other people copy us, and client care for all improves, we have achieved a bigger goal than we could have hoped, although we may have made the hearing aid industry less profitable. We are making top of the range hearing aids more accessible by price, by home shopping, and by audiology services that are delivered over the Internet. We have taken audiology to be 'care in the home'. We also encourage audiologists, and similar professionals, to provide services that address tertiary level hearing care – to provide services that add value, and help those with complex needs. The proportion of people in the community who have hearing loss is rising. If services can be provided in a similar model to that pioneered at Grays Inn Road, then we collectively have some probability of being able to fund hearing health care in developed countries. I want to see audiology practiced at a very high scientific and clinical standard, wherever the practitioner is located.

The client journey today should be: client does the Blamey Saunders SPT online at home. They confirm to themselves that they struggle to hear certain speech sounds and get a medical check of their ears, if possible. Then they order hearing aids. The hearing aids arrive, with initial settings based on the hearing test – the SPT. The client puts on the hearing aids, connected to the programming system, and personalises them further, if help is needed a remote audiology session is booked with us, and we do it for them, or just give advice. As it's a client centred model – the client decides.

But there's much more to come at Blamey Saunders with the Rotary Action Group on hearing, and in helping people to take control of their hearing, and live healthier lives.

Afterthought

Dad was deaf. Mum lived her married life with the sound of silence.

Dad managed his hearing loss very well. He had a very responsible, leadership role in British Rail. He travelled to do international railway projects. But my mother coped with her family, substantially alone. Dad left me with a very strong work ethic; the extreme end of that scale might be workaholic. That can be hard for a partner. So is living with the sound of silence. Dad couldn't hear without his hearing aid, he couldn't hear in the dark, he couldn't hear very well when driving. I didn't think about it much at all. He was just Dad. Researchers have shown that there can be quite a strain on the partner, because communication isn't casual. My dad did his best to hear as well as possible, I have come across many people who don't. I'm campaigning for more awareness about hearing loss, hence starting a company to make hearing more accessible, but as they say, you can take a horse to water, but you can't make the horse drink. When my dad left the house for the last time to go to hospital, even though he was very ill, he made sure he had his hearing aid. I feel a lot of sympathy for people in hospital, or care of any kind, that is cut off from hearing. People need to understand the importance of taking action to hear and the consequences of not doing so. There's no longer a reason in the developed world to put it off. The whole process, from testing hearing to getting on with hearing aids, can be done at home. The next goal is to find ways to help people who still have no solution, because they don't have the means. There are millions of people who have no access to hearing solutions, and where education is much as I descried for 19th century Britain. That's the next project.

Published in 2015 by New Holland Publishers Pty Ltd
London • Sydney • Auckland

Unit 009, The Chandlery 50 Westminster Bridge Road London SE1 7QY UK
1/66 Gibbes Street Chatswood NSW 2067 Australia
218 Lake Road Northcote Auckland New Zealand

www.newhollandpublishers.com

A record of this book is held at the British Library and the National Library
of Australia.

ISBN 9781742576367

Managing Director: Fiona Schultz
Publisher: Linda Williams
Project Editor: Holly Willsher
Designer: Andrew Quinlan
Production Director: Olga Dementiev
Printer: Toppan Leefung Printing Ltd

10 9 8 7 6 5 4 3 2 1

Keep up with New Holland Publishers on Facebook
www.facebook.com/NewHollandPublishers